Blood, Sweat & 2nd Gear
More Medicine for Motorcyclists

Blood, Sweat & 2nd Gear
More Medicine for Motorcyclists

flash gordon, m.d.

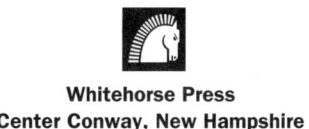

Whitehorse Press
Center Conway, New Hampshire

Illustrations and cover art by Craig Harrison

The medical information in this publication is meant for general educational purposes only and is NOT intended to replace the advice of a person's own doctor.

We recognize that some words, product names and designations mentioned herein are the property of the trademark holder. We use them for identification purposes only.

Whitehorse Press books are also available at discounts in bulk quantity for sales and promotional use. For details about special sales or for a catalog of motorcycling books, videos, and gear write to the publisher:

    Whitehorse Press

    107 East Conway Road

    Center Conway, New Hampshire 03813

    Phone: 603-356-6556 or 800-531-1133

    E-mail: CustomerService@WhitehorsePress.com

    Internet: www.WhitehorsePress.com

ISBN 978-1-884313-63-9

5 4 3 2 1

Printed in the United States of America

Contents

Introduction

If you're immune to illness and injuries, this book's not for you. But if you feel better knowing what's happening when your body isn't working right, c'mon in. In my years as a medical columnist, first at San Francisco's *Citybike Magazine,* and later at *Motorcycle Consumer News,* I've written columns about common conditions, along with tips on how to recognize and (when appropriate) treat them. I've tried to give folks insight into how their bodies work, and how they can go bad. This information is designed to help you avoid the need to go to your doctor, but to understand when that's necessary.

I've been a motorcyclist since 1961, and have been a daily rider more or less nonstop since 1978. I was board certified in Emergency Medicine in 1978, too. Before that, I did my medical school and internship in Miami, Florida, and my emergency medicine residency in Detroit, Michigan (both excellent places to learn about emergencies). I also spent a couple of enjoyable years in Ulm, Germany, as a battalion surgeon for a nuclear missile unit. The emergencies there were relatively minor (thank goodness) but the beer was awesome.

After that, I ran the Emergency Medicine Residency Program at San Francisco General Hospital; worked in various emergency departments; ran the Haight Ashbury Free Clinic's Medical Section; and ended up doing primary care medicine in southern Marin County, California.

I became a columnist for Northern California's famed *Citybike Magazine* in the late eighties, while at the Free Clinic. I've always loved motorcycles, and writing for a motorcycle magazine seemed like a dream come true. I contacted *Citybike*'s publisher, Brian Halton, who liked my work and gave me a monthly column. I was so excited to be in print that it took almost a year before I found out I was supposed to be paid for my writing, after Brian asked why I hadn't submitted a statement yet.

But for me, writing's not about money—it's about the basic meaning of being a doctor. The term "doctor" comes from "teacher" (like a "doctrine" is a "teaching") and giving people useful knowledge really makes me happy (it's like the Chinese proverb "Give a man a fish and he will eat for a day. But *teach* him how to fish and he will sit in a boat and drink beer all day long." Or something like that . . .). By doing my column, I could get useful info to lots of folks at once. And I could also inflict bad jokes on many people, too.

After almost a decade of columns at *Citybike*, Whitehorse Press contacted me and asked if they could put some of my *Citybike* columns together in a book. After I realized it wasn't a vanity press asking me to pay for the privilege of being a Real Writer, I jumped on the opportunity and *Blood, Sweat and Gears: Ramblings on Motorcycling and Medicine* was published. (When I tell my friends in the literary world about this, they always say "The publisher called you??").

After many years at *Citybike*, Fred Rau of *Motorcycle Consumer News* contacted me and asked me to write for them. I was excited about reaching a bigger audience, and have been happily doing an MCN column since 2002. Those columns are the basis of *Blood, Sweat and Second Gear: More Medicine for Motorcyclists.*

I've gone through all those columns, updating the medical information and consolidating them when possible in the interests of clarity. I hope you enjoy them—better yet, I hope the nuggets of medical information help you out. If they do, please tell me; I'm flash@docflash.com. And if you have an idea for a medically-related motorcyle magazine column, please let me know—I'm quickly running out of body parts.

Injuries Caused
by Accidents

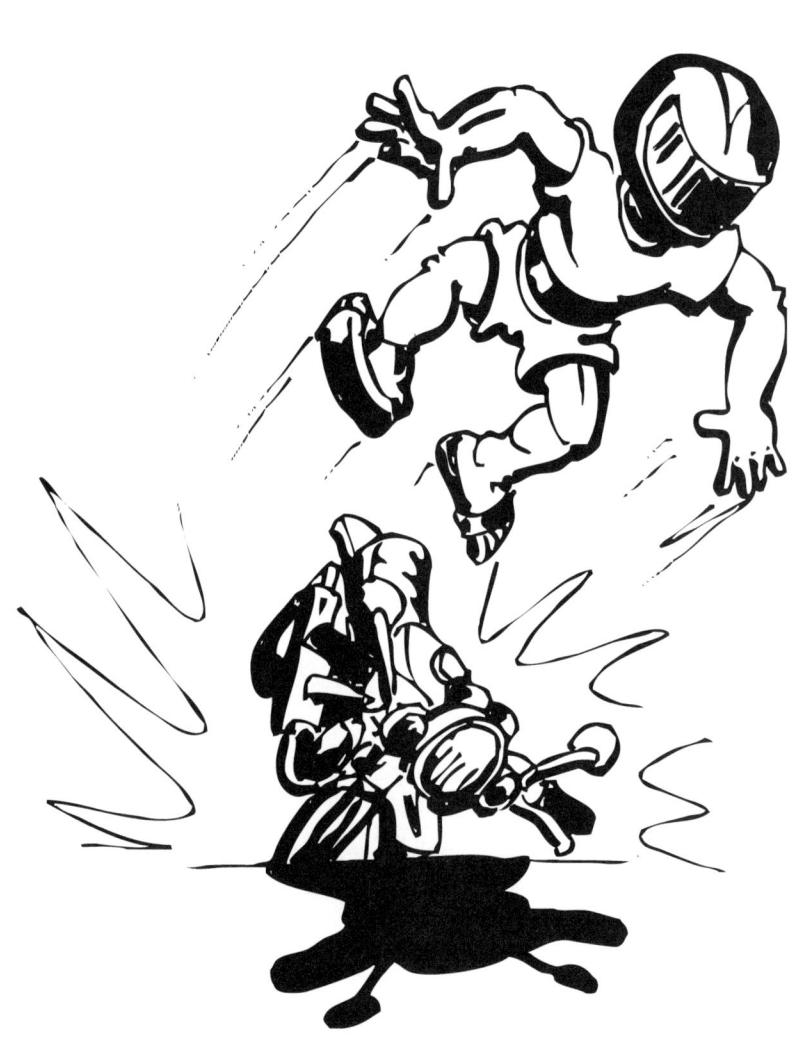

Pavement Dermatitis

Pavement dermatitis (AKA "road rash") affects us all, eventually. Preventing it is easier—and more comfortable—than curing it. In addition to a quality jacket, good riding gear, including gloves, boots, and pants, help a lot. Whenever I see somebody riding wearing shorts, I cringe. Just try crawling on asphalt wearing shorts. Then think of what it feels like at 20mph.

Once you've been scraped, clean it. Betadine®, iodine, and hydrogen peroxide damage tissue. Even plain water is tough on cells. Use a saline solution designed for cleaning wounds (one brand is Shur-Clens®), or saline for contact lenses instead. Saline under pressure is great for removing dirt. In ERs, "squirt gun" type devices or syringes help. Some saline solution comes in squirt-top bottles. Moore Medical, for example, sells 12 oz. bottles for $1.65. But if you don't have saline, don't delay in cleaning it. The faster you remove the germs, the fewer will be there to grow and cause infection. If you can save twenty minutes by washing it in a gas station bathroom, do it.

After the wound is clean, you must remove all the particles of dirt, gravel, asphalt, etc. If left, they'll often stay forever, creating a tattoo. If saline and a sterile gauze pad aren't adequate, try a sterile needle, sticking the dull end into a cork or eraser before sterilizing it. The handle helps.

If you can't get all the particles out, or if you have problems with your immune system or are at high risk for infection, go to your doctor or an ER. Remember, road rash is an emergency doc's bread and butter (I know, not a good image). If you think the wound's deeper than just skin, get it looked at.

Once the wound is clean and dry, the next step is a dressing. In the past, I recommended antibiotic ointments like Neosporin® and some gauze or Telfa®. Here's the problem with this method—though it helped prevent infection, it let the wound dry out, and when the skin on an abrasion dries out, the cells die. This slows down healing. The best way to help abrasions heal is to keep them clean and not dried out. Here's how.

One way is the "semi-occlusive dressing" like Tegaderm® by 3M or Opsite™. These are thin, transparent, adhesive films that are applied directly over the now-clean injured skin. It sticks to the normal skin around the edges of the abrasion, allowing oxygen in and some moisture out. It keeps germs and dirt away from the wound, and helps the skin heal.

Another option is the spray-on dressing, like 3M's Nexcare™ No Sting Liquid Bandage or Medi-Stat™. Spray this onto the *clean* wound, and in 30 seconds it forms a flexible coating. This is great for us motorcyclists, since it's applied with one hand, and works on elbows, knees, and other areas that are hard to bandage. A bottle of this belongs on your bike at all times. Most drugstores have it.

Now, once you've cleaned and dressed the wound doesn't mean you're done. You've still got to monitor it for infection. The four cardinal signs of infection are redness, warmth, swelling, and pain. It's natural to have pain where you've been scraped, but pain that increases in the days after an injury, especially when associated with redness, warmth, or swelling, is an indication that you've got an infection. Another sign of infection is pus at the site of injury.

If you've got a collection of pus under the dressing, it's time to take it off. This lets you inspect the wound more closely for the above signs. The adhesive film dressings like Tegaderm™ or Opsite™ will peel off. The spray-on dressing will dissolve the old dressing. You can spray it on some new dressing and then promptly wipe off (very gently) the old dressing.

Once the dressing is off, clean the wound with more saline solution and look closely at it. A thin reddish border (say, the width of your pinky fingernail or less) isn't that alarming. More redness is cause for concern. It's also worth checking for extra warmth around the abrasion. Here's how to do that.

Touch the area next to the injury with the back of your middle or index finger's middle section. Hold it there for about a half second, and then quickly move it to normal skin a few inches away. Go back and forth, keeping the back of the finger against your skin for about a half-second each time. By doing it this way, you can detect very small changes in temperature. Extra warmth around the wound's edge is another danger sign of infection.

If the wound is getting infected, it's time to contact your health care delivery person. You might benefit from antibiotics.

If you've got a significant full-thickness scrape on the palm side of your hands or fingers, see a doctor. Hands are tremendously complex and intricate structures, and full-thickness skin loss in this area can cause long-term problems. And if you've got a scrape that's right over a joint, be careful. It's easy to get an infection inside the joint itself from a nearby skin injury, even if damage doesn't extend down into the joint.

Joint infections are a serious problem. You can permanently lose use of a joint after only a day or so of an infection. If a joint next to a scrape starts to get more painful when you move it (especially if putting weight on the joint causes pain), have it checked immediately.

After your abrasions have healed, remember that new, pink skin sunburns and darkens very easily. Use an spf 30+ sun block until the pink area matches the skin around it.

And make sure you've had a tetanus booster within the past five years. It is important. I remember complaining to the nurse as a kid in 1961, after an early motorcycle mishap. "Wait a minute!" I said. "Do I really need this? What did people do before they invented tetanus vaccine?"

She said, "They died."

"Oh," I replied.

I got the shot.

Road Rash Decision

I received a letter from Patricia Wilson, a motorcyclist who wants others to benefit from her experience with road rash.

> *I went down on July 4th, 1999 wearing nearly nothing (very hot day that day and I wasn't going that far, uh-huh). I thanked God (and still do) that I have no memory of what happened between the time the front wheel started to go mushy and when I woke up on the pavement. I remember thinking how lucky I was to have this happen this close to University of Michigan's*

trauma-burn unit. I also remember thinking how lucky I was that I didn't lose any skin on my back or butt. It gave me a way to lay without lying on wounds. I had visions of one of those wheel beds.

I don't remember them doing it, but I had a tube inserted in my chest wall to re-inflate the lung that was punctured by a broken rib. It seems strange, but I never had the feeling that I was mortally injured—just injured very badly. When they moved me out of emergency, it was into a trauma-burns unit at University of Michigan Hospital in Ann Arbor. Lucky me; they know how to treat burns. Now I do too, and I think that knowledge should be shared so people have a better understanding of what they are risking when they ride unprotected.

The broken shoulder took about a month to heal. The burns took nearly two years. You get to expand your vocabulary in interesting ways: Eschar, Silvidine, Kerlix, debride, and finally, Jobst. You learn that morphine is great, except for when they come in to 'dress' your burns. You learn that the turnover is fairly high among nurses in trauma-burns because they can't handle the screams. You discover that the friendly cotton washcloth is really woven out of barbed-wire. You learn that this daily process is going to go on not for days or weeks but for months.

I think the worst thing about the daily dressings (gives a whole new meaning to the daily grind) was the anticipation—knowing that the agony you were going through was going to happen again tomorrow and the next day and the next . . . Indeed, it goes on until all of the wounds have completely closed.

Closed, but not healed; for now you graduate to the Jobst garments, which you learn are worn to help minimize (not eliminate) scarring. Depending on where the wounds are, this can be at least uncomfortable. Remember how hot it was the day I went down? Imagine being wrapped in latex fabric in that kind of weather, twenty-four / seven.

Well, in the end, it works. My scars are visible, but not horrific like burn scars used to be, and I did not require skin grafts. It wasn't until five years later that I rode again, but that was mental, not physical. I purchased the bike, the helmet and the summer-weight armored jacket in that order. Speaking of helmets, I examined mine when I got home from the hospital. Had I not been wearing it when I went down, I would have lost a good part of my face to the road.

Patricia makes a good point. Abrasions and burns are similar in the way they damage the skin. A fall at 25 mph results in damage to unprotected skin like that produced by a frying pan containing very hot oil. A faster fall, naturally, produces more damage.

Protective gear makes all the difference. A good set of leathers is probably the best protection available, especially when racing. The problem with them is that riding to work wearing leathers and then changing is time consuming, and more than a little inconvenient. Leathers aren't the best thing in an all-day rainstorm, either. That's why many motorcyclists who spend lots of time in the saddle—touring and commuting riders, for example—often wear fabric suits like those from Aerostich (www.aerostich.com) and Motoport (www.motoport.com). They've got the advantage of

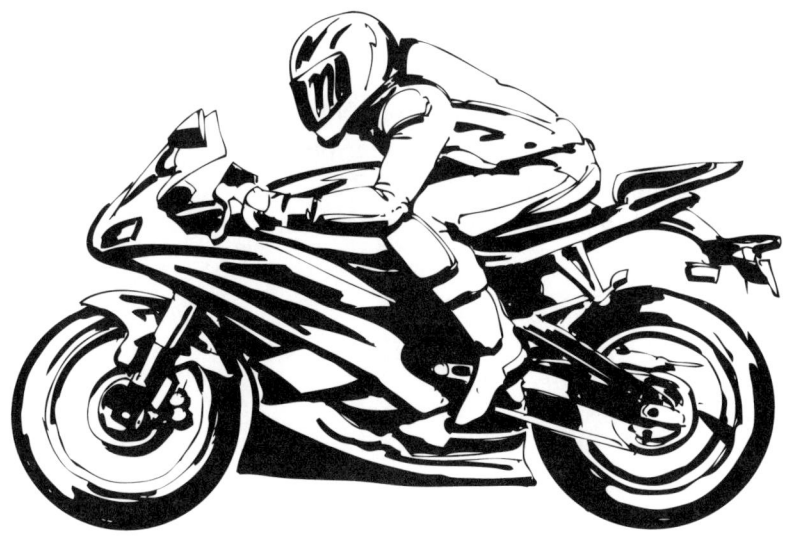

either being inherently waterproof (Aerostich) or have available zip-in liners (Motoport). And the big advantage of these types of suits is that they fit over your everyday clothing.

For folks who want to ride in jeans and a denim jacket, Bohn Body Armor (www.bohnarmor.com) has armored underclothing that fits beneath your outerwear or long-sleeved t-shirt. Though it's less protection than full leathers, it's enough to save your skin.

In hot weather, perforated and mesh jackets, like those from Vanson (www.vansonleathers.com) and Joe Rocket (www. joerocket.com) among others provide substantially more protection than a T-shirt, and are almost as cool.

In the event you do get "road rash," there are some circumstances where going to the ER is especially important. Abrasions over joints, for example, can easily spread infection into the joint itself. And an infected joint may stop working permanently after only a day or so of an infection. Abrasions over bony points (knuckles, ankles, etc.) carry the danger of a bone infection (osteomyelitis). Road rash on the face may lead to permanent scarring, or if there's any dirt in the wound, to permanent tattooing.

Abrasions on the hands (especially the thick, specialized skin on the palm side) should be treated at an ER. Improper care can lead to contractures and loss of use. That's why I always wear good gloves. I find that deerskin, like that from Thurlow (www. thurlowleather.com) and Lee Parks Design (www.leeparksdesign. com) is tougher than leather and more comfortable.

Patricia Wilson sums it up with:

> *I hope you consider writing about this. I think it was David Hough who said, "When you go down, you will be wearing what you decided to wear when you got on." Please help people make the right decision.*

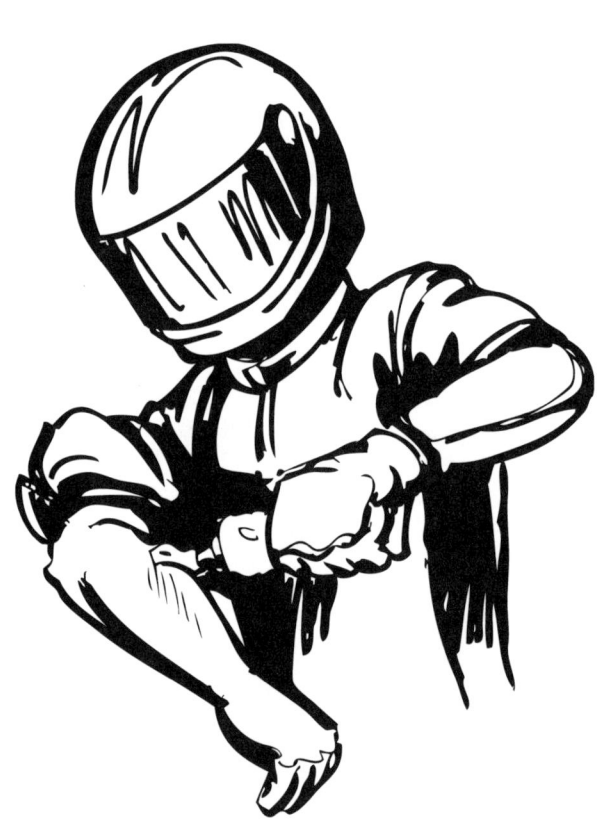

Skin Infections

We all get cuts, scrapes, and burns. And although they usually heal well enough on their own, occasionally they get infected.

Infections can be serious. Most can be treated with antibiotics nowadays, but the germs are getting more resistant. What's worse, they can pass this resistance to other germs, like kids passing a "cheat sheet" during a quiz. The germs are gaining on us.

Any break in the skin can get infected. You can get an infection from a tiny puncture, splinter, or scratch. Injuries that damage a lot of skin, such as road rash (pavement dermatitis) or a burn, get infected more easily. Even some burns that don't initially break the skin, like the one I got from a hot muffler while adjusting the damping on my old stock shocks while my Ohlins were in getting a rebuild, can cause an infection when the blister pops a few days later.

Infections are more of a problem for some people. If you're diabetic and your blood sugar isn't under good control, your white blood cells can't fight the germs as well as they're supposed to. If your immune system isn't working well, either because of an illness like HIV or from medications you might be taking, you're also at higher risk for infection.

You don't always get an infection when bacteria enter your body. There are several factors involved, including your body's resistance to the particular bacteria, the number of bacteria, and how aggressive (virulent) they are. Anything you do to tip the equation in your favor makes it less likely a given injury will get infected.

Since you can't do much to affect your body's resistance, besides keeping illnesses like diabetes under control, and you don't get to pick the germ that enters your body, the only thing you can modify is how many bacteria are in the initial invasion force.

The most important thing you can do to prevent infections is to clean a new injury as soon as possible to remove germs, kill whatever germs are left, and then keep other germs out. It also helps to try to kill any germs that get left in the wound. That's what antibiotic ointments like Neosporin and Polysporin are for.

Next time you get injured, whether it's road rash, or a cut, scrape, or burn, get it cleaned immediately. If you can stop in a gas station, use running water to wash the wound well. Just the movement of the water will dislodge many germs. Keep in mind that *time is critical*—every minute you wait, the germs are multiplying. If you've got water with you, rinsing a new injury immediately, and then doing a more thorough job when you reach running water, makes a lot of sense.

Once you've removed all the germs you can—and that includes removing any visible particles of dirt, rock, or other grunge—applying an antibiotic ointment helps tremendously. This is time-sensitive, too. That's why it's good to have at least a small first-aid kit with you whenever you ride.

After the wound is as clean as you can get it, and it's been slathered with an antibiotic ointment, you need to keep more germs out. That's where the dressing comes in. Dressings need to be changed daily, so you can look for signs of infections. Big wounds, or wounds on the hands, feet, or genitals, are best seen by a physician. It may be necessary to treat them with antibiotics to prevent infection.

It's easy to tell when a wound gets infected. It gets red, warm, swollen, and tender. Sometimes there's pus (dead white cells) or a yellowish crust (impetigo). After an infection has gone on for a while—as little as several hours—it can start spreading in the body. When it spreads into the tissue around the wound, it's called cellulitis. If it spreads though the lymph channels, there'll be a red streak seen moving toward the heart. This is called "blood poisoning," or lymphangitis.

Once you reach the stage of lymphangitis, you'll need antibiotics, in my experience. Hot soaks and rest of the area help, too. Heating an infected area has several good effects. It increases blood flow, carrying more white blood cells and antibiotic to fight the infection. It also speeds up the bacteria, making them suck up the antibiotics and die faster. It also makes your white blood cells work quicker to eliminate the bacteria. In short, it puts the whole process on fast forward.

If you've just got a little infection starting, say, on a fingertip, you can often prevent it from getting worse by frequent soaks in hot water. But once the infection is spreading into the tissue or lymph channels you need antibiotics.

Try not to move the infected part. When you move it, tendons are sliding in and out of the infected area, letting germs hop on the tendon and get past the "perimeter" your body is setting up. One hand surgeon I knew used to say, *"Everything heals faster, when it's put under plaster."*

He liked to cast hands to keep them from moving as they healed. He'd have a window over the infected area to check progress, of course. But if you have an infection somewhere and use that part a lot, you'll slow or prevent healing.

Feet are a particular problem. If a patient has stepped on a nail or has punctured their foot, I put them on antibiotics. If the nail punctured the shoe before going into the foot, I may use a stronger antibiotic (like Cipro). I'll often tell them to stay off the foot for a day or so. Once an infection starts deep inside the foot, patients may need hospitalization for intravenous antibiotics, elevation of the foot, and complete bed rest. Staying off the foot for a day and using early antibiotics may prevent this.

When it comes to infections, "an ounce of prevention is worth a pound of cure."

Band-Aids

Butterfly
Closures

Benzoin Swabs

Disinfectant

Elastic Bandage

Gauze Pads

Combine Dressing

Tweezers

Non-Stick Gauze

Film Dressing

Goop

Wire Splint

Cold Pack

Roller Bandage

Tape

Space Blanket

Triangular Bandage

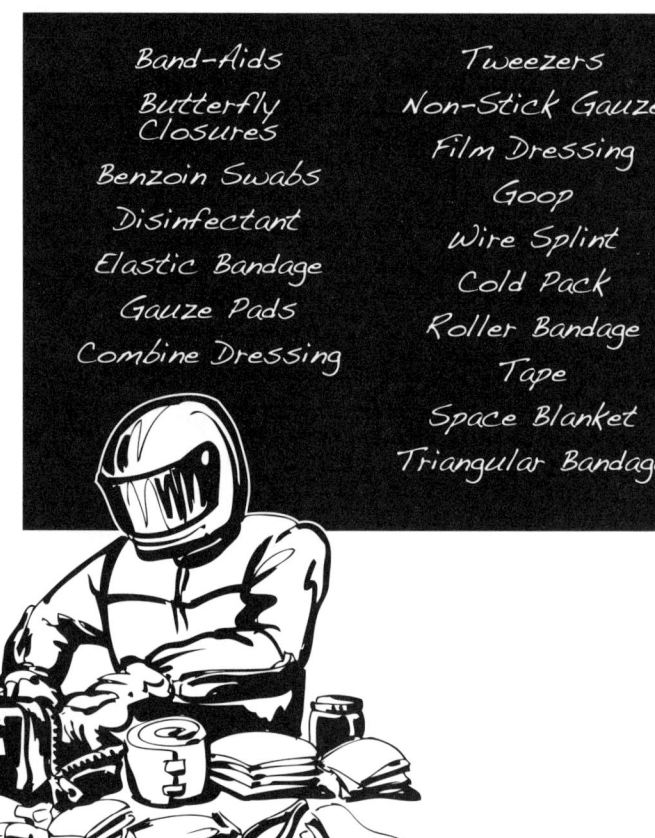

First Aid, at Last

Do you need a first aid kit? That depends. Do you ride mostly in urban or suburban areas, or do you find yourself more than 15 minutes from an urgent care center or an ER? If you're in the first group, just stick some adhesive dressings and antibiotic ointment in your tool kit. If you're in the second group, you'll need more than that. Here are some suggestions on what makes sense to me.

If you're on a trip, you might want to carry all of the items below. Don't forget your prescriptions, carried in their original bottles. If you'll be crossing a national border, it doesn't hurt to carry a copy of the original prescription, too, especially for narcotics or other controlled substances. Hint: Carrying a copy of your glasses prescription is sometimes very helpful.

Gas Station Bathroom One of the essential ingredients in motorcycling first aid. After your next case of road rash, stop at the first bathroom you see and wash the area with running water to remove dirt and germs. If it's not deep, you can use some soap, too, to help sterilize the injury.

Band-aids Band-Aids® are one brand of adhesive bandage, and are sold by Johnson and Johnson. The best adhesive dressings are the flexible kind, which bend with you. Several brands are waterproof, too. The "Coverlet" brand adhesive bandages come in assorted shapes, including knuckle, fingertip, and rectangular (including large ones)—highly useful. When you buy flexible adhesive dressings, it's worth making sure they're latex-free, since, when damaged, skin is more likely to develop an allergy (and latex causes lots of allergy problems). Remember, though, that putting a dressing over a wound that hasn't been disinfected is like giving the germs a shelter.

Butterfly Closures Useful for holding edges of wounds together after they've been cleaned out. They're basically strips of adhesive with a narrow area in the middle that goes over the cut.

Steri-Strips are somewhat similar—quarter- and half-inch work best.

Benzoin Swabs Benzoin helps adhesives stick much better to skin. Note: Don't get it on a scrape or cut—it stings.

Disinfectant Povidone iodine (Betadine®) is what I use. It doesn't sting like the old-fashioned iodine or mercurochrome, and is more effective. Get a pint bottle and keep it at home in the kitchen, where you keep your first aid kit (What? You keep it in the bathroom? When was the last time you got cut or burned in the bathroom?) and just carry a small bottle with you.

Elastic Bandage Often called Ace® wraps (a brand name), they're useful for wrapping sprains, immobilizing fractures (along with a splint), keeping ice packs on sore areas, and for holding gauze dressings in place. A 3-inch wrap is the most useful size (good for wrists) but, if you have room, take a 6-inch, too (for knees). Some elastic wraps are self-adhering, like Coban®. These are handy, since they're less bulky than Ace® and can be used to wrap an ankle and still wear your boot.

Gauze Pads It's worth carrying some 4 x 4-inch gauze pads (called "four by fours" in the med biz—just don't try to buy them in a lumber yard) for use in covering burns, abrasions, wounds, and for cleaning injuries. Bring more than you think you'll need—at least a half dozen. Be sure they're sterile and individually wrapped.

Combine Dressing Often called abdominal dressings, they're big, highly absorbent sterile pads (typically about 5 inches by 9 inches)—good for big wounds.

Tweezers I think Uncle Bill's Sliver Grippers tweezers are the best. They fit on a keychain, and are the best thing I've found for removing splinters. Available from www.slivergripper.ca. Hint: Don't get splinters wet (i.e., with Betadine®) before removing— they swell up. Clean the wound after the splinter's out.

Non-stick Gauze Best known brand is the Telfa® pad. It can be used on abrasions, making removal less painful the next day. Adaptic® is also useful.

Film Dressings Op-Site®, Bioclusive®, TegaDerm®, and PolySkin II® are various brands of transparent semi-permeable dressings. They keep wounds dry (you can shower with them), but allow moisture to evaporate. They're great for road rash (after it's been cleaned, of course) since they maintain a moist environment that promotes faster healing.

Goop Actually, antibiotic ointment. Triple antibiotic ointment, Neosporin, and Bacitracin all are effective. Get whatever's cheapest, and wrap it in something so vibration doesn't rub a hole in the side and cause it to leak all over the place. Don't ask me how I know.

Wire Splint A very useful item to have if you'll be out in the boonies. It's just a piece of heavy-duty chicken wire that you can fold into a splint and wrap to keep fractures from moving. You can make your own, but be careful of sharp edges. They're usually carried folded up.

Cold Pack Putting ice on a new sprain / strain / fracture is a good way to prevent pain and shorten healing time. Cold packs are the next best thing. You squeeze them to activate, and they provide almost instant cold.

Roller Bandage Kerlix® is a well-known brand, and works better than a plain roller gauze because it's stretchy.

Tape I like the clear perforated tape. It holds well, even when wet, and lets the skin breathe. Good for holding gauze in place.

Space Blanket Indispensable for keeping an injured person warm, or for keeping the sun off. They fold up smaller than a pack of cigarettes.

Triangular Bandage Just a big piece of cloth, useful for slings, bandaging, dressings, or pads. Practice using at home, first, and don't forget the safety pins.

Together, all of the above weigh about a pound, and fit into a space the size of a paperback book. Also, call the Red Cross to locate a first aid course if needed. Remember, when it comes to first aid, experience is the worst teacher. It always gives the test first and the instruction afterward.

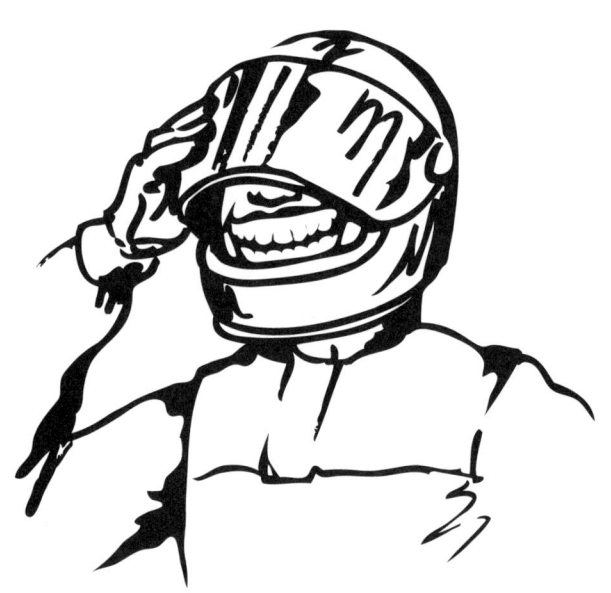

Saving Face

Those folks who always ride wearing full-face helmets might not need this information. Those folks who wear open face helmets (or worse, those ridiculous beanies), pay attention. The face you save may be your own. But keep in mind that face injuries, though dramatic, may be associated with more serious problems, like a broken neck. Other injuries may take precedence.

When I worked in the ER, it wasn't unusual for a patient to come in with a tooth in his hand that had gotten knocked out in an accident. The most common question was "Can you put it back, Doc?" The answer—no. If it was in their hand, it was dry, and if it was dry, it was dead.

Teeth are alive, and once they're dead, they're gone. If your tooth gets knocked out, keep it moist—by doing so, there's a much better chance that it can be replanted. Remember, teeth that are re-implanted in the first 30 minutes have the best chance of surviving. Also, be sure not to handle it by the root. Touch only the enamel part, or crown.

Best thing to do is to very gently rinse off the dirt (don't scrub it—the soft layer of tissue on the surface of the root must be kept intact) and then try to put it back into its socket. If you can get it back, go to the dentist or ER immediately. If it won't easily go back, and the person who's lost the tooth is wide awake and cooperative, he can hold it in his mouth between the gum and the cheek. Don't do this if the victim's got other injuries that might be distracting, or if they're not completely alert and awake. If they're not capable of carrying it in their mouth, put it in milk, saline, or the patient's saliva (not water). A dried out tooth dies within minutes.

Sometimes teeth are loosened a little bit in an accident, but are still in their sockets. If they're only a little bit loose—i.e. they move only slightly with pressure—they'll likely heal by avoiding using them (no biting—soft or liquid food only) for a couple of weeks. If they're really wiggly, a dentist or oral surgeon can fix them in place long enough for them to heal.

The teeth aren't the only things to get injured on the face, of course. Another very common injury is a cut in the upper or lower lip, often caused by a tooth.

When these cuts go all the way through the lip—and it's easy to tell by just holding your lips together and blowing so you puff out your cheeks (air will leak from a through and through cut)—they definitely need to be stitched up. These wounds should be sewn up no more than 12 hours after injury (it's six hours for wounds on parts of the body other than the face) to minimize the chance of infection. Most wounds on the face resist infection pretty well, since the face has a great blood supply, but through and through wounds of the lip or cheek are contaminated with saliva, which has lots of germs.

When these wounds get sewn up, the doctor should sew the inside first, and after that clean the wound from the outside, trying to remove as many of the germs from the saliva as possible. After the wound's been cleaned, the doctor should sew up the flesh and then the skin. If she sews up just the outside, germs from the inside of the cut can cause an infection, preventing good healing.

Another common injury is a cut that goes through the border of the lip—that is, through the line that divides the colored skin of the lip and the normal skin of the face, called the "vermilion border." In these cases, it's critical that the doctor sewing up the lip gets that border perfectly aligned. If it's even a tiny bit off, it's very noticeable. And since lips and eyes are responsible for expression, they're looked at a lot. Even a tiny problem there is very noticeable.

This reminds me of a patient I had back when I was running the Emergency Residency Training Program at San Francisco General Hospital back in the seventies. A woman came in after a bicycle accident. Nothing major, but she did have a cracked wrist and a cut through her lip that went through the vermilion border. She was really attractive, and I didn't want to take a chance that one of the medical students working in the ER would do a less than perfect job. So I said to her "I'm going to call the plastic surgery service, and tell them that you're a professional model. Just play along." She nodded.

I called the plastics resident and explained that she really needed his special level of expertise, since we docs in the ER weren't as accomplished at doing the level of work this "professional model" deserved. He came down and looked at it, and she played along perfectly—she said she did lots of "lipstick modeling," etc. He was so impressed he took her up to the operating room and used an operating microscope to put her lip back together—it looked great.

The crack in her wrist was minor—just a small greenstick fracture of the radius. The intern working on the orthopedic service came down, looked at the X-ray and said "This looks pretty simple. I can just put a cast on it down here." He then asked her "What kind of work do you do?" She glanced over at me, and then said (with a straight face) "I'm a professional pianist."

He took her upstairs and had the attending physician put on the cast instead.

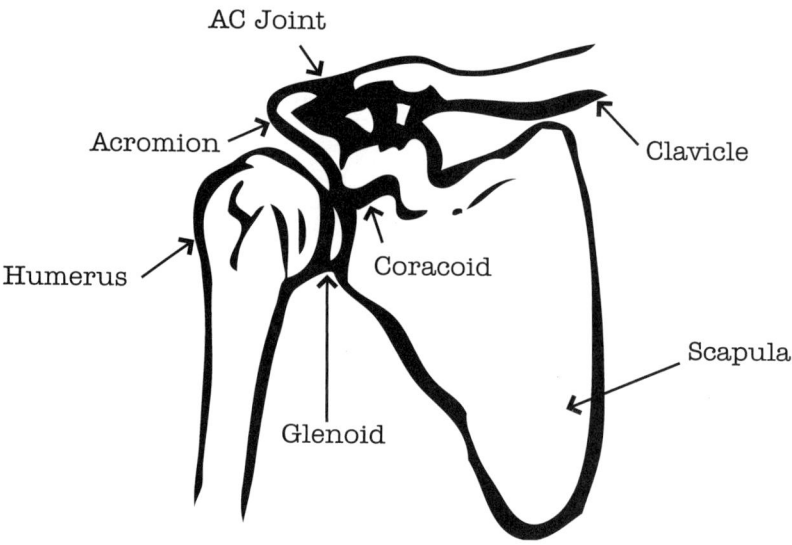

Shoulders

If you have a shoulder problem, raise your hand. Ouch! Okay, my bad. Reaching overhead is hard with many shoulder problems. Let's talk about shoulders and just what can go wrong with them.

The shoulder joint contains three bones—the clavicle (collarbone), humerus (upper arm) and scapula (shoulder blade). The clavicle stabilizes the shoulder, lifting it out and away from the rib cage. The scapula supports the humerus (the ball at the top of the upper arm) in a small hollow called the glenoid fossae. The glenoid is small in order to allow the arm to move in all directions. Some anatomists have compared the humerus sitting on the glenoid to a ball balanced on a seal's nose.

The highest point of the shoulder (go ahead, feel it now) is a part of the shoulder blade called the acromion. If you feel it, you can trace it back down into the shoulder blade. If you move inward toward the base of your throat, you travel over the clavicle. Now, move your elbow in a big circle, and feel the acromion move while the clavicle stays still.

The junction between the acromion and clavicle is the acromioclavicular joint, or AC joint. The muscles used to rotate your arm include those in the rotator cuff, which also help keep the humerus in place. There's a lip of cartilage around the glenoid called the labrum. It provides some stability, too.

Shoulder problems often happen after an acute injury (like an accident) or from overuse (like painting the ceiling). But it's important to remember that not all shoulder pain comes from the shoulder. A pinched nerve in the neck can cause it. But right now we're going to discuss traumatic shoulder injuries—such as AC separations, clavicle fractures, shoulder dislocations, and acute rotator cuff injuries.

One of the most common shoulder injuries is called an AC (acromio-clavicular) separation, which involves straining or tearing the ligaments that keep the outer end of the clavicle attached to the acromion (See the picture). An AC separation can happen when you fall and land on your shoulder. Though many AC separations get better by themselves, some of the more serious ones may need surgery.

In an AC separation, the AC joint (that's the junction we felt earlier between the clavicle and acromion) is tender. Sometimes, the clavicle on that side is higher than the other one. If so, it's because the ligaments connecting it to the coracoid (see picture) are torn. These separations can be more serious, and definitely need checking out. If only the AC joint is tender, there's full shoulder motion, and the clavicle isn't higher than the opposite side, I might just prescribe a sling for a few weeks.

Landing on your shoulder can also give you a fractured clavicle. When broken, the clavicle is very tender, and not shaped like the opposite one. You'll feel a tender bump at the break. A clavicle strap or a "figure eight" dressing helps. You should know how to make one.

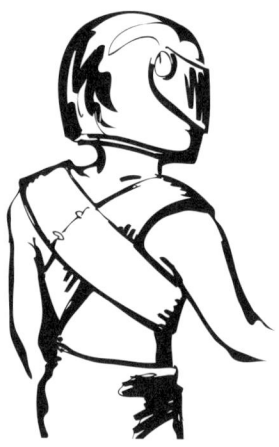

A figure eight dressing pulls the shoulder backwards, so it doesn't put pressure on the broken clavicle, which is what causes most of the pain. To make one, start in the mid back, and then go over the top of the shoulder, down through the armpit, back up and over the opposite shoulder, down through that armpit, and repeat. The shoulders should be pulled backwards, thus taking the pressure off the broken clavicle. If you're 20 miles down a dirt road and your buddy falls and breaks his collarbone, this can come in very handy.

Another common shoulder injury is a dislocated shoulder, which happens when the ball at the top of the humerus slips off the glenoid. Almost all dislocations are "anterior"—that is, the ball of the humerus is in front of the glenoid, and you can usually feel it there. When it's dislocated, you can't touch the opposite shoulder with the hand of the dislocated one. After dislocation, getting it back in place before the muscles cramp is helpful. Though real medical care is preferable, here's a useful "in-the-field" technique.

This self-reduction method is fast and quite often successful. To do it, you sit on the ground, and bend the knee on the dislocated side 90 degrees. Clasp both hands around the knee, then tilt your head upward and lean backwards, pulling the arms forward. Hold this position while relaxing the shoulder completely. The shoulder should pop back into place as the muscles relax. This self-reduction method is fast and quite often successful. After reduction, the shoulder needs a few weeks in a sling to "tighten up" the rotator cuff and capsule.

The rotator cuff is another commonly injured part of the shoulder. It can tear after a fall or collision, and is more likely after being weakened by chronic tendinitis. Tears cause weakness and pain, and it's often difficult or impossible to raise your arm over your head while holding it straight out to the side. Imagine holding a full can of beer in your hand (keeping the elbow straight) and raising your whole arm until the can's over your head. This motion is painful or impossible with rotator cuff tears. They also can cause popping or clicking sounds in your shoulder, which, left untreated, may lead to arthritis.

There are several options to rest an injured shoulder. You can buy a shoulder immobilizer in a drugstore, or use a sling with a band to keep your wrist and upper arm next to your body. Anti-inflammatories like ibuprofen and naproxen help, and ice benefits acute injuries.

Acute injuries, like a broken clavicle, dislocated shoulder, or AC separation usually heal well. More often, folks end up with chronic problems from repetitive injuries, like rotator cuff tendinitis, impingement syndrome and bursitis, or from partial rotator cuff tears that cause arthritis. Don't tolerate chronic shoulder pain. It might get much worse.

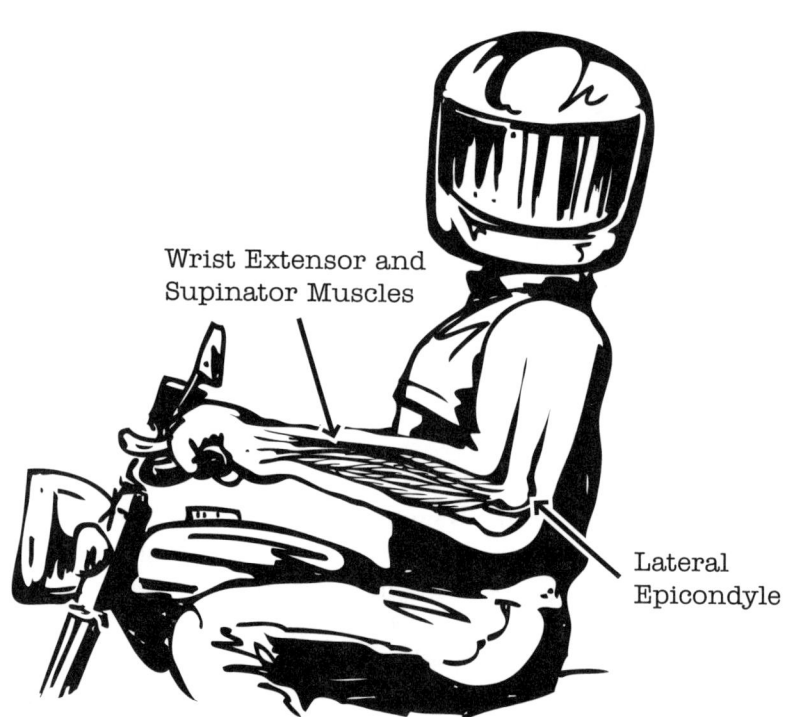

Wrist Extensor and
Supinator Muscles

Lateral
Epicondyle

Tennis Elbow

The medical name for tennis elbow is "lateral epicondylitis." Grab your right forearm near your elbow and bend your right wrist backwards—you can feel the wrist extensors that attach to the lateral epicondyle (the bump on the outside of the upper-arm bone at the elbow) working. The supinators, which also attach there, rotate the hand from palm-down to palm-up. People use them if they are inserting a corkscrew with their right hand. Overuse or injury to the tendons that attach these muscles to the bone results in tennis elbow.

The most common cause is repetitive motion. Repeatedly hitting tennis backhands incorrectly can cause the condition. Pulling something really, really hard (such as lifting a fully-loaded BMW R1100RSL motorcycle that just tipped over, without removing the loaded saddlebags and top case) can also cause tennis elbow. Please don't ask how I know this. (Note: see tinyurl.com/8h2u for the right way to pick up a bike.)

More people get lateral epicondylitis from work than from sports. Usually, individuals who get tennis elbow from work notice pain in the afternoon. It often occurs at that time of day because their shoulder muscles get tired, and they compensate by using the smaller forearm muscles. Some individuals are around 30 years old when they first get tennis elbow, but the condition is most common in those who are over 40 years old.

The pain from tennis elbow usually goes from the elbow down toward the hand. It's often uncomfortable to grip a large object, as you might when holding a cup of coffee without using the handle. This is called the "coffee-cup sign." Picking up thick objects like a big-city phonebook can hurt, too, as can shaking a person's hand.

If you start experiencing this type of pain, find out if it's tennis elbow. If it is, and it's not treated promptly, the condition may become chronic and will be much harder to cure. How do you know if you have tennis elbow? Here are some simple tests.

To do the "middle finger" test, hold your arm in front of you with the palm down. Keeping the fingers straight, push down on the middle finger with the opposite hand. If this reproduces the pain, you may have tennis elbow.

The chair test is accurate and easy to do. Stand behind a small chair (a dining room chair works well—don't try this with a lounge chair) and hold the top of it with your hand facing downward. Try to lift the chair with that one hand. If it causes lateral elbow pain, you have tennis elbow.

Once you have the condition, it's extremely important to treat it properly and promptly. Your best chance for a complete recovery is to start treating it in the first few months. If you don't, you may have it for the rest of your life. Since you use this area for many common hand motions, continued use delays or prevents healing. If it hurts, *don't do it!* For example, when you lift a container of milk out of the refrigerator door by its top, you're using your extensor muscles. If you had a hot case of tennis elbow, you couldn't do this without lots of pain. It's very important to avoid the activity that started the pain, which might mean a change in what you do at work, or eliminating other activities.

There are numerous treatments for tennis elbow. Physical therapy, including ultrasound, is helpful, and should be first-line treatment. Most physicians recommend or prescribe NSAIDs (non-steroidal anti-inflammatory drugs) such as ibuprofen or naproxen, which cool the area and reduce pain. These are really helpful in cases that start suddenly (such as lifting a bike the wrong way). It's not clear if NSAIDs actually help healing. Some physicians think inflammation actually helps initiate healing, and discourage anti-inflammatory use.

Initially, ice the painful area and gently stretch it. Put your arm out straight in front, palm down, and pull the fingers back toward the armpit. You should feel a gentle stretch (not too hard). Repeat this four or five times daily for several minutes.

If you can bend your wrist completely up and down painlessly after a week, start very slow, gentle exercises. Use an 8-oz., filled plastic water bottle as a weight, and hold it palm down. Repeatedly raise and lower the bottle. After several days, gradually increase the repetitions and weight, but do so very slowly. Ice the elbow after the workout. You might feel a little sore, but if the elbow flares up, hold off on the exercise.

If not better in a month or two, an injection of cortisone-type medication (steroid) may often be helpful. Sometimes, though, the effect of cortisone is only temporary, and repeated injections can weaken tissue, leading to rupture. One study shows that individuals who get steroid shots improve more in the short term, but those who only get physical therapy do better in the long run.

A tennis elbow brace can also be useful. It is a strap that goes around the forearm near the elbow, and may help healing. It also reminds you to avoid activities that may be painful.

Acupuncture has helped some people with this problem, as has ESWT (extra-corporeal shock wave therapy—see www.sonorex. com). Controlled studies show mixed results with both therapies.

Surgery is the last resort for tennis elbow, and shouldn't be considered unless you've tried physical therapy, steroid injections, and maybe acupuncture or ESWT. Most surgeons won't operate unless it's a chronic case that has resisted other therapies for six months to a year. Many individuals have very good results from surgery, and more surgeons now use an arthroscope (a surgical instrument that allows surgeons to see and do work inside a joint) for these procedures. It's often possible to return to work within weeks of the surgery.

Another treatment for tennis elbow is injection of the patient's own blood into the spot where the tendon's not firmly attached. The theory is that the localized inflammation as the body cleans up the blood can also cause the tendon to heal tightly, curing the problem. I've had this done to my own elbow, and it worked (for about 3 years). If you (or your orthopedist) are interested, read about it at pubmed.gov—the article is by Edwards and Calandruccio. Just search for "tennis elbow blood injection Edwards."

The bottom line is: If you think you might have tennis elbow, don't ignore it. The earlier the treatment, the better the results. And if you've got chronic tennis elbow, consider asking your doc for a "shot of blood."

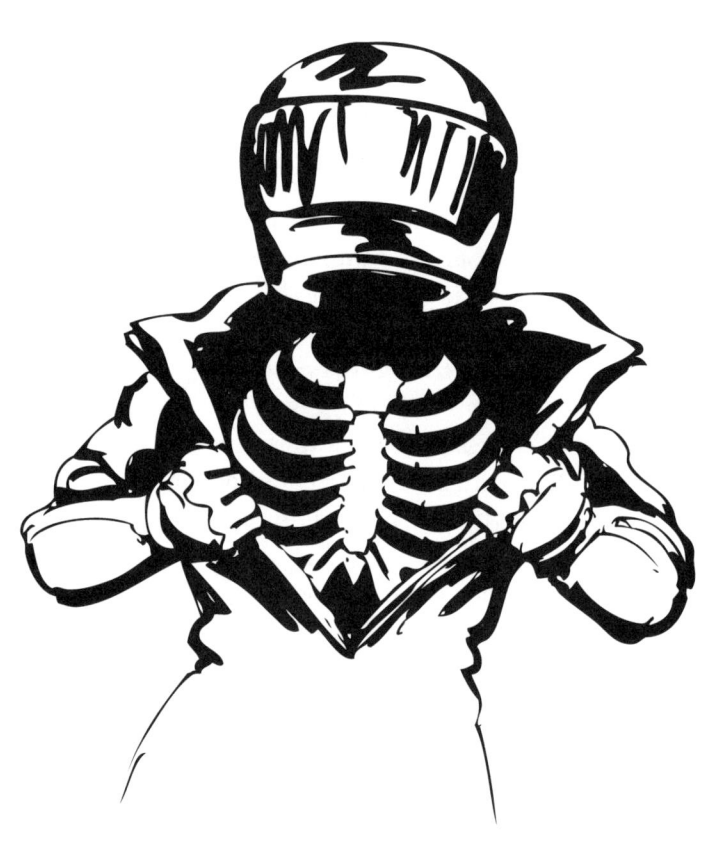

Ribs

Ribs are for more than barbecue. Ribs are part of the bellows that pump air in and out of your lungs. They've got joints where they're attached to your back, and flexible areas where they're attached to your breastbone. This allows your chest cavity to expand and contract, which pumps air in and out. You breathe in when the muscles between your ribs, the intercostal muscles (they're the meat attached to barbecue ribs) pull the ribs closer together, making them more parallel. This moves them upward, and closer to a horizontal position, which increases the chest volume. This sucks in air. When you exhale, you relax, and the weight of the chest wall helps it empty without your having to do any more work.

Ribs aren't that strong. It doesn't take much to break one—step on a pork sparerib some time to see what I mean. A one-rib fracture is more an annoyance than a danger, though in theory it's possible to puncture a lung or other internal organs. The problem with a single broken rib is usually just pain, and an increased chance of bronchitis or pneumonia from under-ventilation.

If three or more ribs in a row are fractured, this danger goes way up. With this much damage, it's harder to keep air moving in that lung and the resulting poor ventilation can lead to collapse of the tiny air sacs in the lung tissue (atelectasis). This is a target for infection.

To prevent the lung from collapsing, you need to inflate it periodically. You can do this with a balloon, a rubber glove, or by just pursing your lips and creating some back-pressure as you exhale, pushing as hard as you would when blowing up a balloon. The increased pressure inside your airways then pushes open the air sacs (alveoli) in your lungs. Do this at least every hour or so after a rib fracture or other significant chest wall injury. If you wait until a cough develops, it's too late. Remember that opiate painkillers, like codeine, hydrocodone (Vicodin), or oxydone (Percocet) suppress your cough reflex. You may start to get bronchitis or pneumonia and not know it until it's too late to prevent.

How do you know if you fractured a rib or just bruised your chest wall? Well, it's easy with an X-ray machine. But you can still often tell if a rib's fractured in the field—here's how.

The ribs form a flexible circle, joining the spine and the breast-bone (sternum). If you hold the sternum in as the injured person inhales, this distorts the circle, causing a cracked rib to bend at the fracture. This hurts. A bruise, on the other hand, usually doesn't hurt. Holding the injured person's sides while s/he breathes in often hurts a cracked rib, too.

A particularly dangerous kind of rib injury sometimes occurs when a few adjacent ribs are broken in two places, keeping the section between the breaks from moving properly. What's worse, when the expansion of the rest of the chest causes negative pressure, the floating section moves inward, which hurts the chest's ability to pull in air. Think of an accordion with a big hole in the bellows, covered with a really loose piece of Saran wrap. When the accordionist pulls the sides apart to suck air in, the patch gets sucked in, too. When the accordion's squeezed, the patch bulges out. The bellows can't move air as well.

In people, this is called a "flail chest," and requires immediate emergency medical attention. When you're calling EMS or the MedEvac helicopter, be sure to use the magic words "the victim is having trouble breathing." You'll get the fastest possible help. In the field, the best treatment is preventing the flail segment from moving. Putting a rolled-up jacket against the broken segment helps. Have the person lie with the flail side down—this keeps it from moving as much.

Treating one fractured rib—as long as you're 100 percent sure that there's no other injury—doesn't usually require MedEvac or an ambulance. It's a good idea, though, to get it checked at an ER just to be sure it's not worse than it seems. Since the motion of the break causes pain, keeping that area still can help keep it from hurting. A "rib belt," which wraps around the chest, can help, also. Taping or strapping works the same way. Though this helps control pain, there's a real danger in this technique. The lung under the break doesn't move well, so it's even more important to use the lung inflation techniques mentioned earlier. The last thing in the world you want is bronchitis or pneumonia with a bad cough, if you have a broken rib or two.

Not all rib problems are fractures. Where the rib joins the sternum, there's an area of flexible cartilage that allows the rib to move. It's possible to damage or to inflame this area. When it's hurt after an injury or direct trauma, it's called a costochondral separation ("costo" means rib, and "chondral" refers to cartilage). When the area becomes inflamed, it's called "costochondritis" ("-itis" means inflammation). Costochondritis can happen post injury or after overuse. Typically, it's very tender when you push right over the area where the ribs join the sternum.

Like rib fractures, costochondral separations take at least three or four weeks to get better. A rib belt, strapping, or taping can be used as a temporary means of support, and it's just as important to keep the lungs well inflated, as mentioned above. Medicines like ibuprofen (Advil, Nuprin, Motrin) are helpful, but a stronger pain medicine is sometimes needed at first.

If there's no separation, but only inflammation, anti-inflammatory medications are usually all that's needed, though a rib belt or strapping occasionally helps. I don't prescribe strong pain medications for this kind of condition.

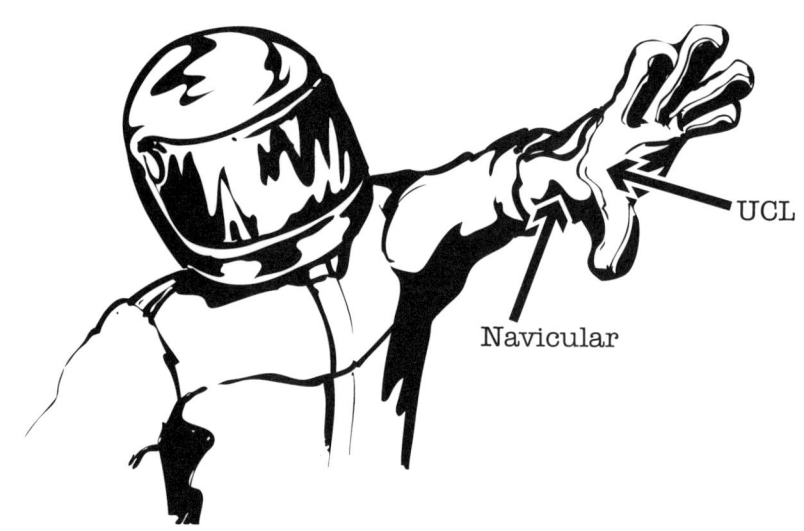

Don't Miss This!

There are lots of possible injuries. Some are treacherous and easy to miss, causing significant disability if not treated properly and promptly.

The most commonly missed fracture on motorcyclists is the navicular bone in the wrist, which results from falling on your outstretched hand. Often, it's not visible at first on X-ray, and is treated as a common sprain.

The navicular supports the metacarpal bone going to your thumb. If broken, pushing your thumb toward your wrist hurts. There's often tenderness in the "anatomical snuffbox." Forcibly twisting another person's same hand inward against resistance hurts, too.

If a patient has a possible fractured navicular that isn't seen on the initial X-ray, I'll splint the wrist and thumb for two weeks, and repeat the X-ray. If I'm still suspicious after a negative second X-ray, a bone scan may help.

It's important to recognize this fracture because the navicular's blood supply isn't great. If not immobilized initially and treated properly, part of the bone can lose its blood supply and die, leading to loss of wrist function. Sometimes, surgery is needed to attempt to correct this. If you fall on your outstretched hand, and have pain as described above, it's a fractured navicular until proven otherwise. Get it checked promptly. A delay in diagnosis could lead to permanent damage.

Another injury not to miss is tearing the ulnar collateral ligament (UCL) in the thumb, also known as "gamekeeper's" or "skier's thumb." If you put your index finger on the web between the thumb and index of the opposite hand, you'll feel the MCP joint (metacarpal-phalangeal joint) of the thumb. The UCL is on the inside of this joint. The MCP is a hinge joint, and isn't designed to go side-to-side. The UCL keeps the thumb from bending away from the index finger. It can get torn in a motorcycle accident if your bike hits something and the handlebar pushes your thumb backwards.

If you tear the UCL and don't get surgery in time, the joint may never be stable. You wouldn't be able to pinch between your thumb and forefinger. If you have pain when trying to pinch forcibly, or tenderness in the above area after a fall or an accident, get medical attention. Don't wait a couple of weeks to see what happens.

When seen, you'll probably have an X-ray. If this shows a fracture where the UCL attaches to the thumb, you'll be referred to an orthopedic or hand surgeon. It's sometimes necessary to pin the fracture for a good result. If the X-ray doesn't show a fracture, it's important that the examining doc test the ligament to see if it's looser than the other hand's. Testing the ligament is done by gently bending the thumb sideways, which may be painful enough to require an anesthetic injection.

Another injury that can cause catastrophic results if missed is compartment syndrome. This one can lead to the loss of an arm or leg—or even death.

Your arms and legs have "compartments," which are areas where the muscles are enclosed within a membrane, called the fascia. If blood is added to this compartment, pressure can increase to the point that blood flow to the muscle is cut off—just as you'd get from having a tourniquet on the limb. Note that having a pulse in the limb does not rule out compartment syndrome, since the higher pressure in the artery may carry blood through the compartment, but the pressure can keep blood out of the tissue. Timing is everything in compartment syndrome—in severe cases, you may start to have damage in as little as 4 to 12 hours.

There are a few signs of compartment syndrome to watch for. Pain that's more than you'd expect from the degree of injury is the most common and most significant sign, which is why too much pain medication right after an injury can be dangerous. Other signs include pain on stretching the muscles of the limb; numbness or tingling (paresthesias); and increased pressure in the compartment (the arm or leg will feel more "tight" or "tense" to fingertip pressure). Occasionally, pulse will be decreased or absent, but *this is not reliable*. Of course, if the pulse goes away, there's a Big Problem.

One cause of bleeding into a compartment in a limb is a fracture. When this happens, the doc taking care of you is more likely to consider compartment syndrome as a possible complication. If the fracture is casted immediately, swelling may occur inside the cast. If pain is increasing after the cast is applied, and especially if the pain is throbbing, you should not delay in having the cast split (bivalved). In some cases, this is all that's needed to reduce pressure in the compartment, allowing blood flow. A 3:00 a.m. visit to an emergency room for this purpose is completely justified—and not going might cause permanent damage.

However, if the bone's not broken, but some muscles are crushed and partially torn, that can be enough to cause compartment syndrome. If they bleed enough to increase the compartment's pressure to the point that blood won't flow into it, that can cause the muscles and nerves to die. Other causes include gunshot wounds, stab wounds, insect bites, infections, and electrical injuries. Almost anything that causes swelling in a compartment can cause compartment syndrome, even simple overuse.

Treatment is simple—the compartment is opened surgically under anesthesia. This procedure is called a fasciotomy, since they cut the fascia enclosing the compartment. This relieves the pressure, and if done promptly, can save the limb. If not done in time, muscle breakdown products can clog up the kidneys and cause renal failure, and in some cases death may result from heart rhythm problems. Other complications can be permanent contractures of the muscles involved, as well as possible amputation of the limb.

If you or a companion have any signs of the injuries we mentioned here, get seen promptly and ask the doctor "Ulnar collateral ligament? Navicular fracture? Compartment syndrome?" Riding a bike is much easier with an even number of arms and legs.

Potential Troubles
on the Road

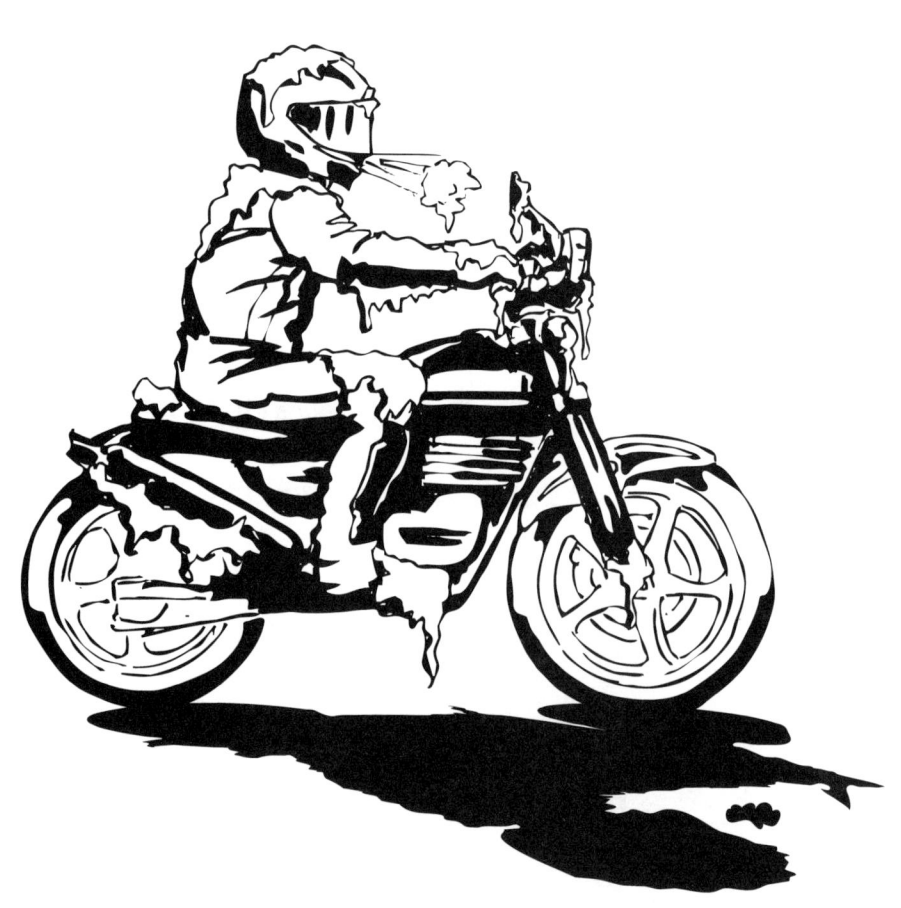

Hypothermia

Hypothermia is Latin for "low temperature," and happens when your body loses more heat than it can make and keep. Hypothermia causes loss of judgment, impairs concentration, and decreases blood flow to your extremities. Next, your hands and arms stop working well, which is not recommended while riding.

Poor judgment is an *early* symptom of hypothermia, making it tough for you to recognize there's a problem. As Alan Watts said, "Trying to know your own mind is like trying to bite your own teeth." The subsequent loss of coordination, strength, and concentration is a potentially lethal combination.

Preventing hypothermia is much easier and safer than reversing it. All heat loss is by either convection, evaporation, radiation, or conduction. You can control all four.

Convection is heat that's picked up by the air. When Mother Nature blows on you when it's cold out, it's called "wind-chill," which cools you faster than just the air temperature would suggest. More air moving picks up and steals your heat faster.

Evaporation cools you, too, so stay dry. "Cold and wet" is the opposite of "warm and dry." Riding in cold rain when unprepared can be lethal.

Radiation causes you to lose heat constantly if your clothes are cooler than your skin. And if you have a fever, you'll lose body heat a lot faster. Remember that, if you ever need to ride when you're ill and it's cold outside.

Conduction happens when you're in contact with a colder surface. A good base layer like polypropylene helps prevent this, since it acts as a good insulator, even when damp. Damp cotton doesn't insulate.

Your body can get heat either from within or from outside. Your metabolism and your muscles create heat. Shivering is your body's way of turning up the "idle" on your muscles to increase heat production. Although shivering helps, using big muscles makes more heat. If you're cold, stop, do some squats, step up and down on a curb, or take a short brisk walk.

You can also "import" heat from the outside. Electric clothing is a great way to ride safely and more comfortably in the cold. But remember that a cold wind on the outside of your electric vest will carry that heat away. A windproof layer is vital.

To reduce losses, think of how you're losing your heat. Clothing keeps heat in. Lady Godiva was *not* ready for a winter ride. Leather or textile riding suits minimize convective heat loss, especially on a bike without wind protection. If you've never worn leather or windproof textile pants along with your jacket, you'll be astonished at how they'll extend your comfort range.

Insulation prevents conductive losses as temperatures drop. Zip-in insulating liners help, as does a fleece jacket under the windproof shell. An electric vest or jacket can provide you with great amounts of heat, allowing you to be comfortable and safe in below-freezing temperatures. Long underwear keeps warm air next to your skin, cutting convection, radiation, evaporation, and conduction losses.

Polypropylene is an ideal material for cold weather riding, both next to the skin and when used for layering. It insulates well when damp, unlike cotton, and it wicks moisture away. Stopping for gas and going inside might make you sweat when dressed for the cold. Sweaty cotton is cold. Polypropylene wicks away the moisture and keeps you warm.

I've skied in a snowstorm (not good riding conditions) wearing a polypropylene fleece jacket without a waterproof shell. At lunch, I found the fleece was literally soaking wet. I wrung cups of water out of it, but I was warm. That same fleece jacket lives in my tankbag on most trips, and is comfy around a campfire or in a restaurant.

Handguards in front of handgrips help a lot, since your hands lose heat fast in the wind. And once you've experienced electric handgrips, they become more of a necessity than a luxury, since they *add* heat to your body through your hands. Good gloves are critical in cold weather, since your hands and fingers act like radiator fins. In a pinch, a pair of cheap dishwashing gloves worn over your riding gloves can help a lot—they'll keep the wind off your hands, reducing convective loss. Snowmobile-type hand covers make cold weather rides safer and more comfortable, and are now being made specifically for motorcycling.

The latest technology in gloves is "phase change interface" material, as used in gloves made by BMW and by Lee Parks Designs, among others. They're expensive, but I think the wide comfort range and excellent feel in my Lee Parks Deerskin PCI gloves is worth it.

Even your engine heat can help prevent hypothermia—my BMW twins' jugs warm my feet. In a pinch, you can warm your hands on the engine—but be sure to wear gloves, avoid the exhaust pipes, and be extra careful if both hands aren't on the bars. It would be safest to stop the bike if you decide to warm up using the engine.

In a pinch, wrapping newspaper around your legs and chest under your clothes helps. I got caught in the fog in Mendocino, on the Northern California coast one summer in 1978. It was *cold*. Dishwashing gloves and newspapers saved my . . . umm . . . heat.

Food is vital to keeping warm. You need calories to heat your body. But a big meal diverts blood from your extremities to your gut. Snacking or several smaller meals is a better way to keep up your caloric intake if you're cold.

You need water to maintain your blood volume. When dehydrated, blood gets diverted to your core *from* your extremities, which then get weaker and uncoordinated. Watch your urine—if it's dark yellow, you need to drink more water. If you don't need to urinate every four hours, drink more.

Treating mild hypothermia is easy. Stop, get into a warm place, and have something hot to drink. Walk around, using your big leg muscles. Don't ride until you're warm and aren't shivering. And if you're really cold, and it's getting dark, and you don't have the right gear—stop. A motel room is a lot cheaper than a hospital room.

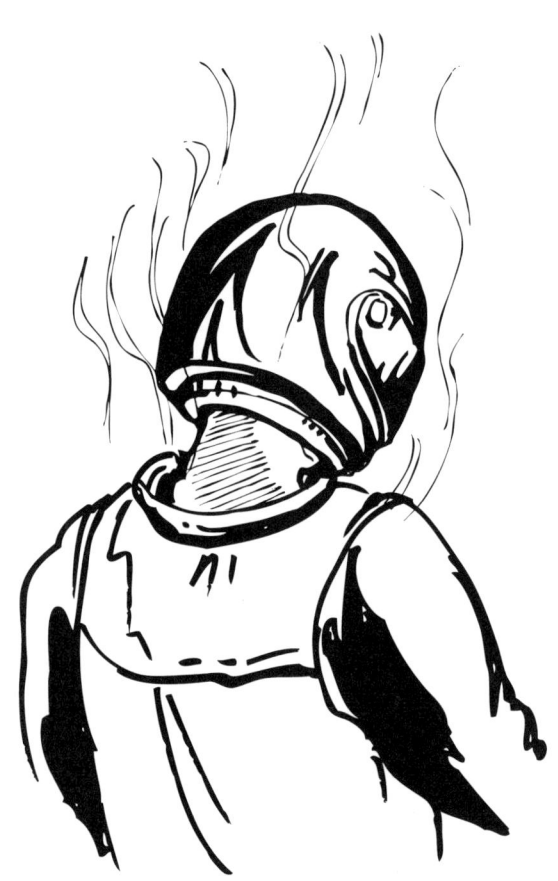

Rednecks

Many motorcyclists are rednecks. It's not where they live, their political views, or how they talk—it's sun exposure. Even when we're fully suited up, the backs of our necks can get sunburned.

Over time, I've learned to put on sunscreen before a long ride. I'll usually remember to do my face. (Hint: Some brands of sunscreen irritate eyes when you sweat and it runs, but Neutrogena brand doesn't do this to me.) However, I'll often forget the back of my neck on the first few days of a trip. By the third day, though, the pain back there serves as a good reminder; but by then, I'm a redneck.

Sunlight causes more than sunburn. It's responsible for aging, too. Sunlight causes about 90 percent of a Caucasian's skin aging. Victorian women used parasols (para = for, sol = sun) to preserve their complexions. That works. Keeping the ultraviolet A off your skin will let it age about 10 percent as fast. So if you keep all the UV-A away from a 32 year old's skin for 30 years until age 62, the skin would look 35. If you're not convinced, take a close look at the skin of your inner arm just below your armpit. See how young it is?

Sunlight is also a major cause of skin cancer, like squamous cell carcinoma (SCC), basal cell carcinoma (BCC), and melanoma. Though localized SCC and BCC are curable, melanoma is often fatal. Since skin cancer is the most common cancer, you need to know what to look for.

Early sun changes are pre-cancerous actinic keratoses (AK). The skin in an AK is thick, often crusty or scaly. AKs are often found on the face, scalp, hands and other areas getting lots of sun. They can turn into SCC. People who drive a lot tend to get them more on the left side, since that side's in the sun.

Squamous cell carcinoma is diagnosed in around 200,000 Americans each year. Like BCC, SCC occurs most often in sun damaged skin, but can show up in skin that's been burned, radiated, or exposed to chemicals like arsenic, or chronically exposed to some petrochemicals. Though it usually stays in the skin, it can metastasize and kill you. It's more likely to spread when it starts on chronically inflamed skin or on mucous membranes, like lips.

SCC usually has a red, inflamed base, and is crusty or scaly. It may present as a sore, bump, or just a crust. Fair-skinned people with sun exposure are at the highest risk. When they occur on the lip, they're more likely to metastasize. Sores that don't heal in a month, that bleed, or that change should be looked at.

Basal cell cancer (BCC) is the most common of all cancers, affecting about 800,000 Americans annually. It's usually on sun-exposed areas, and looks like a shiny bump or nodule. It grows very slowly, and tends not to metastasize to other parts of the body. When it occurs near important structures, such as the eye, it can be treated with a remarkable technique called Moh's micrographic surgery.

In this technique, the surgeon cuts out the tumor and draws a grid on the bottom, and the piece that's removed is examined for cancer cells microscopically. If, say, two squares of that grid still show cancer invasion, the surgeon removes more tissue from those two grid squares. By continuing to "map" where cancer invades, the surgeon can trace it, sparing normal tissue.

Malignant melanoma killed an estimated 7,910 people in the US in 2004, compared to 3,927 on-road motorcycle deaths. Of these, 5,050 were men and 2,860 were women. In 2004, 55,100 new cases of melanoma were found in the US, so the death rate is about one in seven (slightly better than Russian Roulette).

Now, the bad news; recent sun exposure isn't the big melanoma risk, but the sunburn you got in your teens is. One bad sunburn as a teenager doubles your lifetime risk. Lots of freckles or moles, fair complexion, blond or red hair, and a family history of skin cancer also increase the danger of melanoma.

However, not only fair-skinned people get melanomas—people of African background get them, too. 16 percent of melanomas occur in blacks, and there's a strange tendency for them to occur on the soles of their feet. Everybody is at risk.

"Normal" moles you've had all your life can also turn into melanoma, so you need to know the difference. Learning what to watch for is as easy as A-B-C-D-E.

A stands for *asymmetry*. "Good" moles are round, indicating that the cells are growing at the same rate. Cancer cells tend to be "free spirits" and grow at different rates. A melanoma is more likely to have halves that don't match.

B is for *border*. A good mole's border should be sharp and distinct from the unpigmented skin around it. Melanomas often have an edge that's scalloped, irregular, or indistinct.

C means *color*. Good moles are evenly colored. Melanomas often aren't. They even can develop grey, red, white, pink, or blue shades. If a mole's color isn't even, get it checked.

D indicates *diameter*. Skin lesions that grow or are more than 6mm (about the diameter of a pencil eraser) should be looked at.

E means *evolving* or changing. If an existing mole bleeds, grows, itches, or changes, have it looked at.

If a melanoma is caught early enough, it's 100 percent curable. If not . . . Well, remember those 7,910 deaths. Though there are constant advances in chemotherapy, you're far better off finding one before its cells decide to go on a road trip through your body.

Also, don't forget that not all melanomas look like moles. Lentigo melanomas are flat and thin, like a giant freckle. Spreading superficial melanomas can be flat or a little raised, and often have a more uniform color. Sometimes, melanomas occur on the palms and soles, or under fingernails or in cuticles. Occasionally, they'll occur in the eye. The above A-B-C-D-E guidelines still apply.

Remember, skin cancer is the most common kind of cancer. And unlike other forms of cancer, if you keep your eyes open, you can catch it and kill it before it kills you.

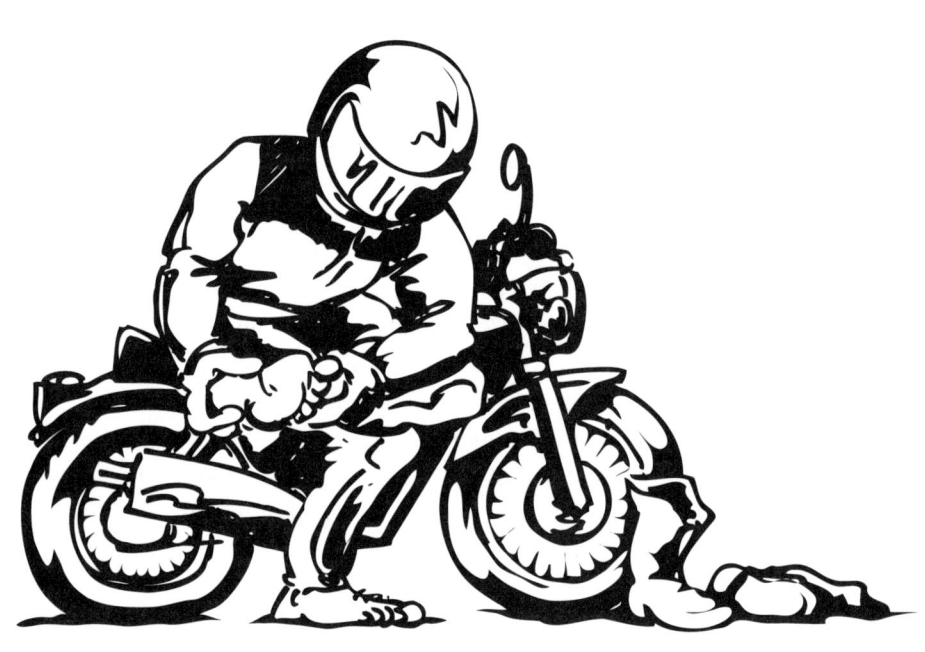

Feet, Don't Fail Me Now

Are your feet jealous of your hands? Probably so, especially if your feet are stuffed into socks and boots all day while your hands are breathing fresh air.

One problem resulting from this confinement is athlete's foot, tinea pedis, a fungal infection. Athlete's foot fungi like dead moist skin; shoes and socks keep skin between toes moist—perfect fungus food.

You first notice athlete's foot when you feel itching between your toes and see cracked skin. At this stage, I recommend buying some miconazole cream (trade name Micatin). It works a lot better than the older Desenex type meds. Put it on twice a day, and don't stop until a week or so after the last trace of athlete's foot disappears.

Remember, athlete's foot itches. It doesn't actually hurt unless bacteria have started to eat the live skin that's been exposed at the bottom of the crack in the dead skin that's been made by the fungus. A good rule of thumb (rule of toe?) is that if athlete's foot starts to hurt, you've got an infection. Infections in the feet can get bad quickly, since circulation in the feet isn't that great. If athlete's foot does start hurting, you should see your doctor. Foot infections can be hard to heal. This is especially true if you've got poor foot circulation, are diabetic, or have immune problems.

Don't try to cure a foot infection (or any infection, for that matter) by smearing it with an antiseptic like Neosporin or Betadine. Putting it on your skin after you've got an infection down in the tissue doesn't do anything. It's like trying to kill bugs in your basement with poison on the roof. The only exception to this rule is a prescription topical antibiotic cream and ointment called mupiricin (trade name Bactroban), which can penetrate the skin, and in some cases will eliminate a superficial bacterial infection.

On the other hand, antiseptic ointments are very good for preventing infections, as long as you put them on the break in the skin right after it occurs. Keep a tube of antiseptic ointment handy if you're going to be doing something that's likely to result in an injury. Putting it on immediately (even if you skip the bandage) is much better than waiting 20 minutes to clean and dress the skinned knuckle.

This principle is worth remembering if you ever find yourself with road rash. Get some antiseptic goop on it as soon as possible, don't wait until you get home. One tip: If you put a tube of antibiotic ointment in your tool kit, vibration will rub through the side of the tube quickly. Wrap the tube in a couple of sterile 4 x 4-inch gauze pads.

Back to athlete's foot: I'm not sure where it got its name, but I have an idea. It probably comes from communal showers, like those in gym class. Fungi lurk on wet floors, and walking barefoot there is a good way to catch it. I used to take flip-flops when I traveled for use in showers, to keep my feet away from athlete's foot fungus spores.

For the last few years, though, I've been traveling with a pair of Crocs, the dorky looking rubbery plastic shoes that look like clogs, often with holes in them (www.crocs.com). They're great shower shoes, being non-slip (originally invented as boat shoes) and antibacterial. Since they're well ventilated, they keep the skin of your feet dry, and make it much harder for fungi to grow, helping prevent athlete's foot. What's more, they're the most comfortable shoes I've ever worn, and are great for your feet and back. They only weigh about 6 oz., and feel great after a long ride. In fact, I keep a pair at my office, so after riding to work, I take off my riding boots and wear the Crocs during the day.

Another common foot problem is toenail fungus, or onychomycosis. It causes nails to get thick, deformed, yellow, and sometimes flaky. It doesn't do any real harm—it just looks ugly. But not only is it ugly, it's hard to treat. The most effective treatment available currently is antifungal pills, like Lamisil (terbinafine) or Sporanox (itraconazole). These drugs require monitoring of liver function, and can interact with many other medications. Not only that, itraconazole may affect heart function. Unfortunately, even when taken every day for three months as specified for toenail fungus, each of these agents has about a one in three failure rate. For many people, it may not be worth taking these medications.

There's a topical treatment called Pen-Lac (ciclopirox) which is safer, but unfortunately it usually doesn't work (not much of a trade-off). However, there are new products in development that are now undergoing clinical trials and look very promising. Unfortunately, they're about three years or so from hitting the market. But if you've got toenail fungus, you might want to try a clinical trial (www.clinicaltrials.gov) to get treated earlier. There are other, non-government trials being held, too.

Another common foot problem is excessive sweating. This may contribute to fungal problems, as well as "stinkfoot." One way to help control it is by appropriate footwear—I'm a big fan of Smart-Wool socks, since they're both very comfortable and do a great job of wicking away moisture. Getting your motorcycle boots off whenever possible helps a lot, too (see previous comments about Crocs).

Folks who need to change socks a few times daily may have a condition called hyperhidrosis (excessive sweating). This often involves the palms, soles, and armpits. There are prescription strength antiperspirants that can help; Botox injections are sometimes useful for armpits; and a technique called "tap water iontophoresis" where a small electric current is passed through the skin while soaking in tap water has been shown to be very effective in controlling sweating and the resultant odor.

Last, remember this: If your feet smell and your nose runs, you're built upside down.

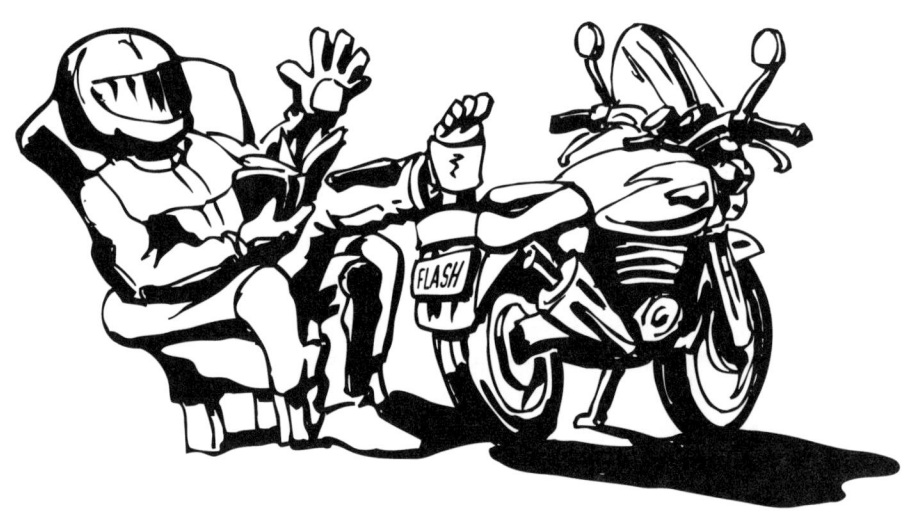

Ouch!

Ever been sore after a long or vigorous ride? Ever sprain something? Here's what you need to know to handle these situations.

The human body contains both hard and soft tissue. Hard tissues, like bones, can break—soft ones, like ligaments, muscles, and sometimes tendons, can get strained, sprained, or torn.

Unlike some motorcycle parts, these soft tissues can stretch for quite a while. Enough force, though, will partially or completely tear a tendon, ligament, or muscle. Less stretching is called a "strain." It usually causes minimal disability. More force will partially tear the ligament or tendon. In this case, we call it a "sprain."

Treating acute injuries of this type correctly is very important. With proper treatment you'll heal faster and hurt less. You can also prevent a partial tear from becoming a complete one. The four components of treating a new injury are Rest, Ice, Compression, and Elevation, which you can remember as RICE. Here's how each of those components of proper treatment work.

Rest allows your body to limit the damage. Typically, when you sprain something you tear some tissue. Torn tissue means torn blood vessels, and torn blood vessels leak. That's why it's common to see a bluish discoloration after a sprain or fracture. You're seeing blood under the skin. If you use the injured part, it'll keep bleeding, causing more pain and slower recovery.

Ice helps by decreasing blood flow to the injured area. Just put some ice in a plastic bag and wrap it in a towel or cloth. Even better is a package of frozen peas or corn wrapped in a towel, since it conforms better to the shape of the injured body part. The resulting decrease in circulation helps slow or stop bleeding in the injured tissue, which means less swelling, less pain, and a faster recovery.

Compression helps limit both swelling and internal bleeding, but you have to be careful. I've seen folks come in after an injury with an elastic bandage wrapped so tight that it has cut off circulation to their hand or foot. If an elastic wrap is causing numbness, it's too tight. Gentle pressure is usually all that's needed to decrease the swelling that results from blood leaking from injured tissue, and from fluid oozing through the walls of irritated blood vessels in the injured area. Here's a tip: If wrapping a sprained ankle, put some cotton or wadded-up tissue paper in the space below the "ankle bone" (medial or lateral malleolus), since that's where the most commonly injured ligament is. Direct pressure on the injured area helps limit bleeding and swelling, making for a faster recovery with less pain.

Elevation helps in the same way. By decreasing the pressure in the veins in the area, there's less leakage and better circulation. Here's a good demo: Look at the veins in the back of your hand, and then raise your hand higher than your head, watching the veins. See how they collapse? That's what happens when your hand is higher than your heart. Less blood in the veins means less blood in the tissues, and less blood = less pressure = less bleeding = better circulation = less pain = better healing. Elevation also helps circulation, since with less blood in the veins, there's more room for arterial blood to enter the injured area.

When swelling starts to prevent blood from freely flowing into the injured area, you'll start to feel throbbing. If you only remember one thing from this discussion, remember this—*Throbbing in a body part after an injury is a Bad Sign.* It means the blood's not getting in where it's supposed to. So if it's throbbing, get it higher than your heart. If the throbbing continues, and the part's getting numb, seek medical attention *without delay.* A 3 a.m. emergency room visit is completely justified.

Muscles can be injured, too, most typically by tearing microscopic muscle fibers. This is normal during resistance exercise, like weight lifting or using exercise machines. You can only build up muscle by first breaking it down through exercise. That's one of the reasons a vigorous workout makes you feel sore—you're feeling those microscopic muscle tears. After a really hard workout, you may even see little bluish discolorations under the skin, which is the tiny muscle tears bleeding.

The other reason for soreness after a workout is lactic acid. Muscles make lactic acid when they need to use more energy than their blood supply permits. Once it's there, lactic acid is painful and can contribute to cramping as well. Stretching after muscle use (including sitting in the saddle all day) is a good way to prevent this. Heating muscles after they've been used helps prevent soreness, too. A hot bath or shower increases oxygen-rich blood flow to the muscles, which helps remove the lactic acid.

Warm-ups and stretches both help prevent muscle pain. The warm-up increases blood flow to the muscles you're about to use, decreasing your risk of injury. Stretches are particularly good too, especially after vigorous activity. If all of a muscle's fibers are stretched, they're much less likely to be sore the next day.

Another hot tip: If you're expecting a really hard day, take aspirin, ibuprofen, or Aleve first. They help prevent inflammation and reduce pain. If you wake up achy, take more the next day with food. Adults can safely take two adult aspirin every four hours if needed for pain; however, ibuprofen or naproxen (Aleve) will probably be easier on your stomach. It's important to always take these with food and a full glass of water, otherwise, you can easily irritate your stomach. And remember to smell the aspirin before using. If it smells like vinegar, it's gone bad. *Don't take it.*

Last, staying in shape (and I'd appreciate it if those of you who know me personally would stop snickering) helps prevent injuries. Ideally, exercise has three components: cardiovascular, stretching, and resistance. Cardio increases endurance, stretching helps prevent injury, and strength makes it a lot easier to pick up the bike after leaving it parked on hot asphalt using the sidestand.

Don't ask me how I know this.

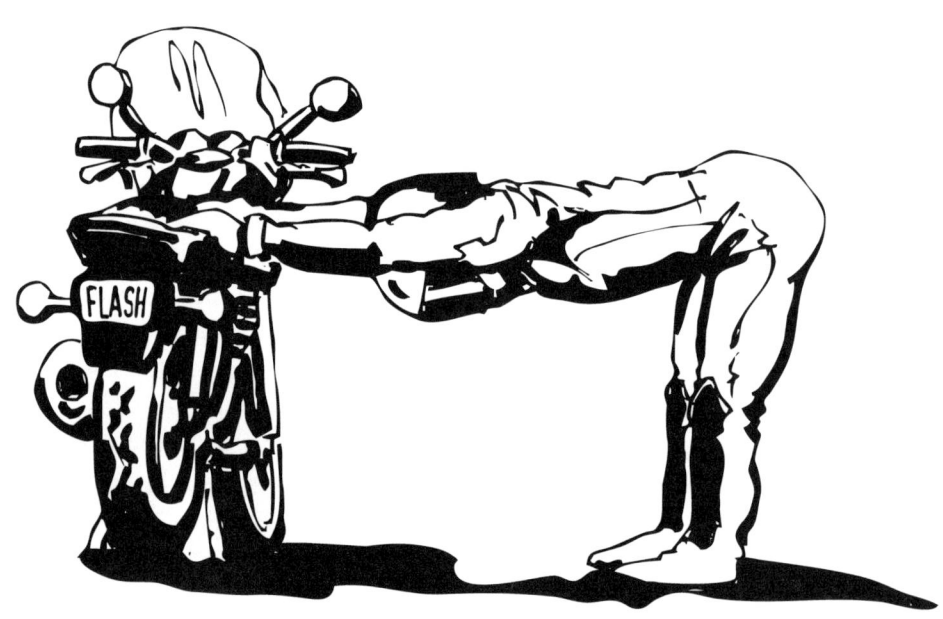

Bend or Break?

Remember the 500cc 1969 Kawasaki Mach III? It was the quickest bike of its time with 12.61-second quarter-miles at 111.38 mph. However, its poor handling killed people. A bike's handling and suspension is like your body's flexibility—just as your strength is like the engine, and your cardiovascular fitness is like the fuel system. You—and a bike—need all three. And though lack of flexibility might not kill you, it can lead to discomfort, sprains, strains, and even ruptured discs.

Flexibility (which you get by stretching) has particular benefits for motorcyclists. In an accident, flexibility prevents injuries. Falling while inflexible is like bungee jumping using a chain . . . *Ouch!* After a long ride, stretching and flexibility prevent aching muscles. Good flexibility helps improve coordination, and we all know what the technical term is for an uncoordinated motorcyclist—an ex-motorcyclist. All these benefits make motorcycling safer and a lot more enjoyable.

Stretching is the best way to develop flexibility. Different techniques have been popular over the years. When I was young, we were taught "ballistic" stretching in phys. ed.; this was trying to touch your toes by "bouncing" a little lower each time. Ballistic stretching caused tiny tears and bleeding inside the muscles, and damaged connective tissue. It could even cause a ruptured disc. Never "bounce" when stretching.

Slow, gentle, and prolonged stretches were the standard after bouncing got bounced. This is still popular and fairly effective. Here's an example using a stretch you've seen runners doing—they look like they're pushing over a building.

Stand at arm's length away from a wall and put both hands on it. Then, put one foot behind you with the heel on the floor. Slowly lean into the wall, noticing how your calf feels. As you lean closer to the wall, you'll feel the calf stretch. Now hold the stretch for 30 seconds or so. This is a "slow and gentle" stretch. Don't stretch to the point of pain. You'll hear the calf complaining some, but *not* screaming.

You're feeling the stretching sensation because of your proprioceptors. They're sensors inside the muscles that feel what position the muscle is in, and that pass that info up to your spinal cord and on to your brain.

Proprioceptive Neuromuscular Facilitation (PNF) uses proprioceptors in a newer and better stretching technique. When you stretch a muscle, one set of proprioceptors signal the spinal cord that the muscle is stretched as far as it's "supposed" to go. Your spinal cord then tightens the muscle, stopping it from getting longer and possibly tearing. You'll also feel a stretch, and perhaps pain, depending on how hard you're stretching. After a few seconds, the spinal cord tells the muscle to relax, which prevents damage from over-tightening. After this second group of proprioceptors fire, relaxing the muscle, you can stretch it more effectively.

Here's how to use PNF to your advantage. Start by stretching the muscle until it starts to feel a stretch. Then, tighten the muscle *without letting it shorten* for 5 or 10 seconds. The stretching feeling should go away. Then relax the muscle, and you'll find that it easily stretches a little further. If you repeat this several times, you'll be able to stretch out a tight or cramped muscle quickly and effectively.

Here's how you'd do a PNF stretch of a calf muscle, perhaps right after a charley horse. Do a calf stretch as described above, leaning forward until you feel a stretch. After about 30 seconds of gentle stretching, gradually push your toes against the floor while keeping the heel down (but without changing your body's position) until the stretching feeling goes away. Don't push with all your strength—just until you *don't* feel the stretch. After 5 or 10 seconds, stop pushing and slowly lean a little closer toward the wall. You'll find your calf stretches farther. Repeat a few times, alternating 5 or 10 seconds of toe pressure on the floor (tightening the calf muscle) with leaning a little farther forward for a gentle stretch for 30 seconds or so.

Don't try to stretch a cold muscle—it's easy to tear and damage it. A cold muscle is like a cold tire—it needs to be warmed up before you can do much with it. The best time to stretch is after you've been using the muscle. It'll be warm and flexible, and stretching will be easier, safer, and much more effective. Also, post-exercise stretching keeps muscles from tightening up. Five minutes of stretching after a long ride helps prevent stiffness and soreness.

Here's a back, hamstrings, and shoulders stretch you can do on the road. Stand on the right side of your bike, with your fingertips against the seat. Bend over so your arms, back, and butt are level, with your knees slightly bent. Gradually lower your shoulders until you feel a stretch. Now gently straighten out your knees until you feel the hamstrings stretch, too. Remember, if you feel pain behind your knees, you're pushing too hard.

To add PNF techniques to your shoulders and upper back stretch, gently push downward with your hands without letting your upper body change position. When the stretch feeling fades, hold it for 5 or 10 seconds, and then relax downward, increasing the stretch some more. Repeat. To PNF stretch your hamstrings, gradually tighten them as you're bent over until the stretching sensation fades. Hold for 5 to 10 seconds, then let your upper body sag downward until you feel them stretching again.

Your forearms benefit from stretching, too. Try putting your fingertips on the handgrips and gradually leaning into them. After 30 seconds of feeling a forearm stretch, push with your fingers (without moving) for 5 to 10 seconds, then stretch again. Remember, don't do this when cold—warm your muscles up first by using them. Same goes for your shoulders and hamstrings. You'll be looser and more comfortable the next day.

Remember—being looser means you're more likely to bend than to break.

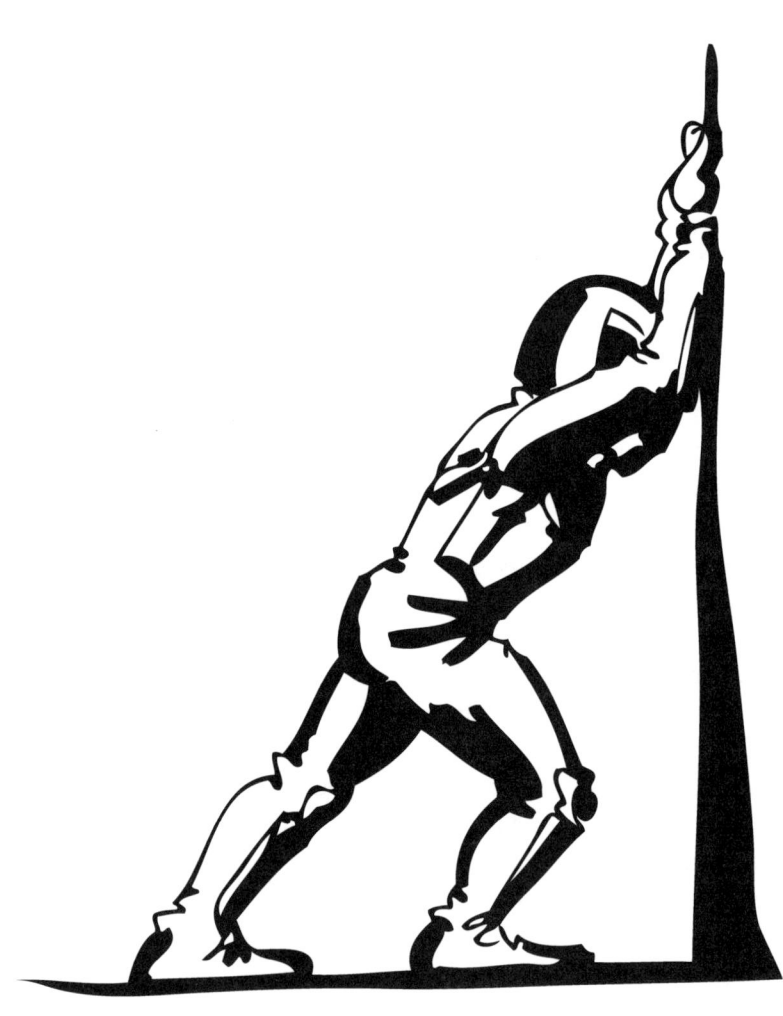

Cramps 101

Cramp. Spasm. Charley horse. We've all had them. They're often in the calf, which is good. It's easy to grab your calf, massage it, and stretch it out by using the foot as a lever. Massage and stretching is the basic treatment for many cramps. Proprioceptive Neuromuscular Facilitation (PNF) that we just discussed is great for some kinds of cramps.

Electrolyte problems and muscle trauma can both cause cramps. Untreated cramps can sometimes spread to surrounding muscles—that's why you might have a twinge in your back on day one, while on day two you can't get out of bed. Stretching after using your muscles can prevent cramps.

An imbalance of electrolytes, which are minerals found in the blood, can be caused by loss of fluid (as in sweating, vomiting, or diarrhea) or by lack of adequate electrolyte input. Calcium, potassium, sodium, and magnesium are some of the common electrolytes associated with cramps. More commonly, dehydration from inadequate fluid intake, or insufficient salt intake, is what leads to cramping. When exerting yourself, or if you're in hot or cold weather, drink enough so you need to pee at least every four hours. If you're not acclimated to the heat, make sure you get enough salt in your food. If you're craving something salty, *eat it.* After a while, in hot weather, your sweat glands start conserving salt—until then, you can sweat enough salt to cause electrolyte problems.

Trauma is another cause of cramps—the kind of trauma you get when you pull a muscle. Overuse injuries commonly cause cramps, too. Picture this: You've just gotten a new GSX-R1100 to supplement the cruiser you've been riding for several years. You decide to ride down to L.A. from San Francisco, stopping only for gas. If you weren't already in good shape, your back might start sending you a message about the time you pass Santa Cruz. That message would be "stop/stretch/relax." Listen to your back.

If you finished the 450 miles to L.A. ignoring your back's advice, you could feel like a steel pretzel by the time you got there. Spending too much time in a new and uncomfortable position can cause this. Your muscles are being stretched and worked in a way they're not used to. Pain, and likely, cramps, may result.

Okay, so you've got a cramp. What do you do? It depends.

If you've been sweating a lot, there's a good chance that the cramp is due to an electrolyte imbalance. Drink a bottle of Gatorade and a bottle of water, if you have them. One way to tell if you need Gatorade or another electrolyte replacement drink is how it tastes. If it tastes really good, you probably need the electrolytes. If a sports electrolyte replacement drink isn't available, eat a meal that has some salt, and drink a few glasses of water. That should help.

If you've pulled and partially torn a muscle and now it's cramping up, use ice and rest, and perhaps very gentle stretching or massage. Be careful when stretching or massaging a partially torn muscle, since that can cause more blood to ooze from damaged muscle fibers, which may make things worse. Taking ibuprofen, aspirin, or naproxen (Aleve) immediately after an injury can make it bleed more, too. If you feel a defect in the muscle, or if you see blood under the skin, don't massage it—just use rest, ice, compression, and elevation. Don't forget to take some Tylenol (acetaminophen) for the pain. Ibuprofen, aspirin, or naproxen (Aleve) would be okay if it's just pulled, but not a torn muscle, since the latter may increase bleeding.

Heat and massage are good for cramps from overuse. Try to find a motel with a hot tub. You'd probably also benefit from a massage. A good, deep, slow, and lengthy massage will push the blood into the tight muscles, and help flush out the lactic acid that causes pain.

PNF (Proprioceptive Neuromuscular Facilitation) is a great technique for relieving overuse cramps, in my experience. This often will stop a cramp immediately, and often prevents its return.

But stretching to prevent cramps works even better. Stay loose.

Numb Hands

Numb hands affect many motorcyclists. Common causes include carpal tunnel syndrome, vibration white finger, hand-arm vibration syndrome, thoracic outlet syndromes, as well as pinched nerves.

When I have a patient with numb hands, I find out what they mean by "numb." To doctors, numb means "asleep"—like your jaw is (hopefully) at the dentist. Most patients, though, call a pins-and-needles sensation numbness.

This sensation is classic for nerve compression. Pressure on the nerve affects its blood supply. Since nerves work by conducting an electrochemical reaction, the lack of blood to that section of nerve interferes with the transmission of sensation, so the nerve transmits a partial signal, which the brain interprets as static, or a pins and needles feeling. Nerve pressure from sitting on the toilet too long, or having someone fall asleep on your arm, often causes this. Though many patients think the tingling is due to poor circulation, it's the poor circulation *to the nerve* that they're feeling.

Numb hands are often due to nerve pressure. The single most common cause is riding with a lot of weight on the wrists while the wrists are bent back. One common scenario is the rider who's been riding a cruiser and has been riding with his hands hanging from the bars with his wrists bent back. Since there's no weight on them, this probably won't cause a problem. But when he buys a GSX-R with its lean forward riding position, he gets numbness after riding for a while. Most likely he has Carpal Tunnel Syndrome.

Carpal Tunnel Syndrome

Carpal Tunnel Syndrome (CTS) is a real problem for riders, since improper hand position and bad riding habits can cause it, or make it worse. Left untreated, CTS can lead to permanent disability or surgery.

In CTS, you may notice your hand or hands getting numb or

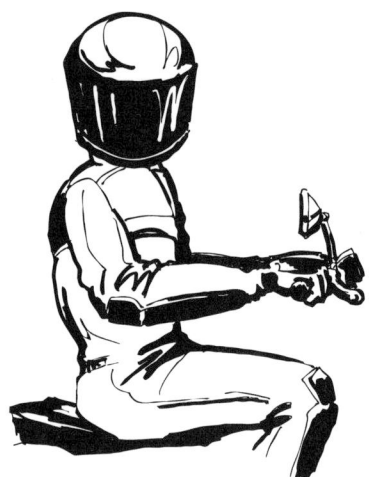 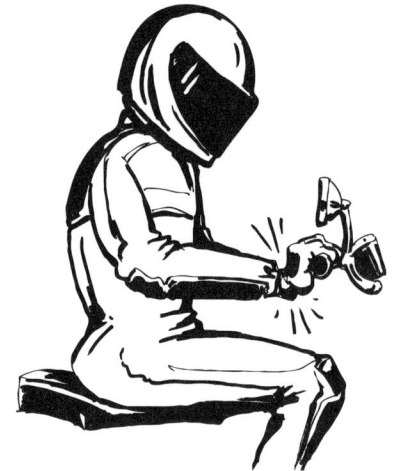

tingly during or after a ride. Sometimes there's pain shooting up the arm from the wrist, or weakness in the hand. You may start to drop things. *Night pain* is an especially important and significant symptom. If you wake up at night with numbness in your hand(s) and find yourself shaking your hand to get the feeling back, CTS is likely. You should see your doctor if you get these symptoms.

How does CTS occur? The carpal tunnel is where the median nerve and some of the tendons to your fingers pass through the wrist area. This "tunnel" lies just beneath the creases on the middle of the inside of your wrist. In this area, the bones form a U-shape with a band or "strap" of tissue across the top of the "U." This band prevents the tendons from bulging out when you bend your wrist forward and grasp. There's not a lot of extra room here, and if things get tight, there's extra pressure on the nerve.

Try this: Straighten out your wrist and fingers so your hand's straight in line with your forearm, as if it were resting flat on a table. Now feel the inside of your wrist where the creases are on the inside of your wrist. Then, bend your hand and wrist back. You'll notice that the inside of your wrist in that area gets harder. This is putting pressure on those structures in the carpal tunnel.

A new injury, like a bad sprain, fracture, crush injury, or dislocation, can cause acute carpal tunnel syndrome or nerve compression. If you've injured your wrist recently and are wearing a splint, cast or even an elastic bandage, watch out for numbness or throbbing, especially in the first day or so after injury or casting. If it isn't relieved by loosening the elastic wrap and/or by elevating the injured wrist, get in touch with your doc as soon as possible. If you've just had a cast put on, an emergency room visit to split and loosen the cast might be indicated.

More typically, inflammation and/or swelling of wrist structures cause the first episode. You may only feel pain or tingling, which gets better. This doesn't mean there's no problem—if you repeat the activity that caused the problem originally, it may recur, and it may be worse. Eventually, if pressure on the median nerve continues, you may get frequent tingling, pain, weakness, or numbness.

Activities that stress the tendons in your wrist over and over are a type of repetitive trauma, and are a major cause of carpal tunnel syndrome. When you use muscles or tendons a lot, they tend to get bigger and stronger. That's okay for your bicep, since it's not in a confined space. However, when the tendons in your carpal tunnel get bigger from overuse, they put more pressure on the median nerve, which also is in the carpal tunnel. This pressure causes CTS.

In the past, the typical patient with CTS was a jackhammer operator. He'd be squeezing the handle of a jackhammer all day, and the repetitive vibrations could lead to swelling of the tendons in the carpal tunnel. Now, most CTS patients are folks who do lots of keyboarding or other data entry (like cashiering in a supermarket). As a rider, you increase your risk if you ride with your wrists bent back while leaning on them. This squeezes the structures in the carpal tunnel, and can lead to CTS. Pregnancy can also cause CTS to develop.

A common test for CTS is tapping the inside of the wrist with a fingertip. If pain or tingling shoots into the hand, it's a sign of CTS.

Treatment for carpal tunnel syndrome can take a long time. There are two types of therapy—non-surgical and surgical. Non-surgical treatment includes aspirin, ibuprofen, or other non-steroidal anti-inflammatory drugs (also known as NSAIDs), as well as rest, stopping the activity that caused the CTS, physical therapy (PT), and wrist splints, especially at night. The splints seem to be very helpful to some patients. If you have carpal tunnel syndrome and haven't tried them, you should. Remember, also, that acetaminophen (as in Tylenol) doesn't have anti-inflammatory effects, and isn't as helpful as an NSAID.

Try to be aware of the position of your wrist. If structures in the carpal tunnel are already swollen, having your wrist bent back will make things worse. Keeping your wrist in a neutral position is one of the big advantages of night splints. It can also remind you not to overstress that wrist.

Surgery for carpal tunnel syndrome is indicated when you've got a hand that's getting worse despite conservative measures like PT, rest, splints, and NSAIDs. If you've got a hand or fingers that are numb most or all of the time, you may be a good candidate for surgery. Surgery might also be needed if you've got an acute buildup of pressure due to a crush injury or a fracture.

Luckily, surgery for CTS is usually very helpful, as long as you haven't delayed so long that the continuing pressure on the nerve has caused permanent damage to it. In CTS surgery the surgeon will usually lengthen the "strap" that goes over the top of the tunnel. This relieves the pressure, and often cures the symptoms and prevents them from recurring.

What can you do as a rider? Try not to put pressure on your hands with your wrists bent backwards. Make sure the angle that your front brake lever and clutch make keep your wrists closer to straight than to bent. Don't tighten your gloves too much around the wrists—that adds to the pressure on the nerve and can make things worse, too. And, you may also find that using bar-backs to move the controls closer can be all it takes to prevent CTS from occurring.

Thoracic Outlet Syndrome

Other parts of the body can cause nerve pressure affecting the hands. The nerves to the hands leave the spinal cord in the neck, exit the torso through the thoracic outlet, and go down the arms. The thoracic outlet is a crowded area. There are muscles, bones, blood vessels, and nerves, all in the same small space. Thoracic outlet syndrome (TOS) affects these structures.

I had a patient who came to me complaining of numb hands. He rode a BMW R100GS, not a sport bike. He rode with his wrists fairly straight, and didn't lean on them. However, he didn't have a windscreen on the bike. Since I know that the nerves that pull the head forward can impinge on the thoracic outlet area, I had him push his forehead against my hand. After a couple of minutes, his hands got numb. When I released the pressure, the numbness went away. The solution? Buy a windscreen. It worked for him.

One test for TOS is the "Stick 'em up!" test. Stand up against the wall with your upper arms horizontal, elbows slightly behind your head, and forearms vertical, palms forward. Your shoulder, elbows, and the back of your wrists should be touching the wall. Open and close your hands slowly for three minutes. If you get symptoms, that suggests TOS.

Another place the nerves can be affected is in the neck. Nerves exit the spinal cord between the vertebrae toward the back. If a person has neck problems, bending the neck backwards can put pressure on the nerves. When riding a sport bike with the body leaning forward, a rider has to tilt his head back. In some cases, this can put pressure on the nerves, causing numb hands. Sometimes a set of bar risers can cure this. They can also relieve wrist pressure, which by itself can add to the problem.

Vibration White Finger

Hand-arm vibration syndrome is a lesser known cause of numbness. Repeated vibration may cause the blood vessels in the hands to temporarily close, causing symptoms. A related condition is called "vibration white finger" which is made worse by cold. Since vibration can contribute to problems like carpal tunnel syndrome, it's important to minimize it when working with a case of numb hands. If vibration's a big part of the problem, bar-end weights or a Bar-Snake can sometimes help. Gel palms on your gloves and cushier handgrips help a lot, too.

The take-home message: If you're getting numb hands, check if they're getting cold and white. If so, the first thing to do is work on minimizing vibration. If they're pink and warm, look at the ergonomics of your ride, such as your head position, wrist position, and whether you need a windscreen. Your hands will thank you.

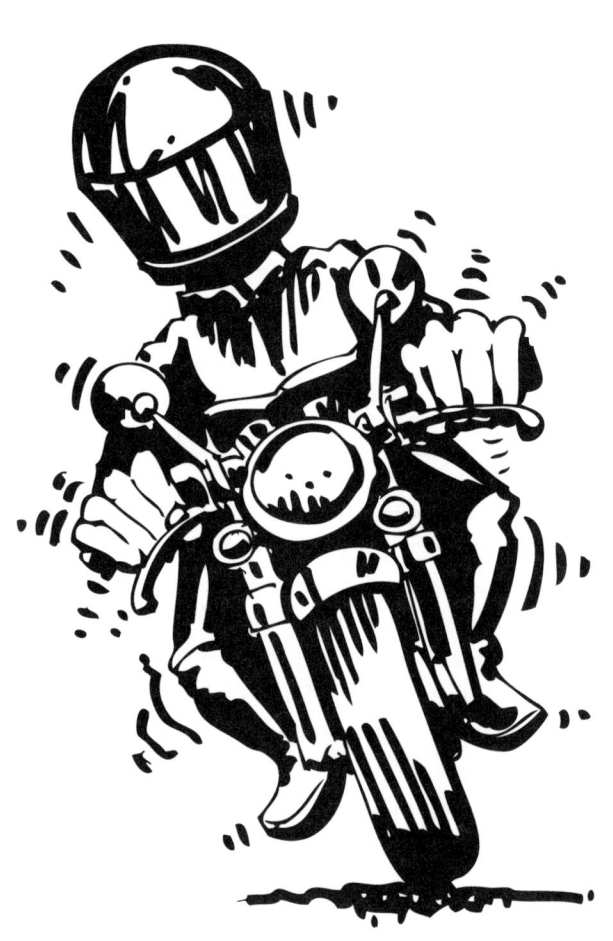

Bad Vibes

People chronically and repeatedly exposed to vibration are prone to a condition known as "vibration white finger" or sometimes "cold finger" (no relation to Gert Frobe). The more modern name for this condition is "hand-arm vibration syndrome" or HAVS. It was one of the most common work-related conditions in the industrial world, until recently, after workers comp claims skyrocketed.

One research study looked at car mechanics in Sweden, whose main exposure to vibration was using pneumatic wrenches on lug nuts, averaging 14 minutes per day. The 806 mechanics had, on average, work experience of 12 years. About one in four had symptoms of HAVS or of persistent numbness, and 40 percent of those who'd been exposed to vibration for 20 years had neurological findings upon examination.

This problem is more common than most people realize. Among workers, almost one in ten who work with vibrating tools may suffer from HAVS. However, since manufacturers and employers are becoming more aware of the problem, steps are being taken to limit the exposure of workers to vibration, and this problem is on the decrease. Motorcyclists, though, may vary widely in the amount of vibration they're exposed to and how long they experience it.

What does this mean to motorcyclists? Obviously, some of us are at higher risk than others—those who ride more, those whose bikes vibrate, those who hold the grips tighter, and those of us who've been riding for a longer time. Luckily, there are things that reduce the risk significantly. First, though, you need to know what to watch out for.

A cold, white finger is often the first symptom. In normal fingers, blood supply is reduced somewhat, but not completely, with cold exposure. In folks with HAVS, blood flow to the fingers may stop entirely, giving them a cold, pale finger or fingers, possibly with numbness or pain. As the oxygen in the finger gets used up, the finger may turn blue. After rewarming, fingers may redden, tingle, and/or hurt. Nerve damage can result, eventually causing permanent numbness and/or muscle weakness of the hand and forearm. In advanced cases, the problems may persist for many years, even after exposure to vibration stops. There is no known cure—only prevention.

Smokers are about twice as likely as non-smokers to get this problem. This is probably related to the decrease in blood flow caused by smoking, and possibly due to the lowered oxygen levels associated with the carbon monoxide in cigarette smoke. Which do you like better—your fingers or your cigarettes?

Exposure to cold increases the risk of HAVS. It's just as important to keep the body core warm as it is to keep the hands warm. When riding, good gloves aren't enough to keep your hands warm—you'll be astonished how long underwear can improve the quality of your ride, if you don't wear a riding suit or leather. I've found heated grip kits indispensable, as has every rider I've known who's tried them. They're available for under $30 online (tinyurl.com/5KSU), highly recommended, and they fit under regular grips.

People who are stressed a lot, for whatever reason, are more susceptible to HAVS. This makes sense, since stress hormones decrease blood flow to the extremities. Decongestants, some migraine medication, amphetamines, cocaine, and even caffeine have been known to trigger problems. Keep this in mind if you ever have HAVS symptoms. Also, beta blockers like propranolol, atenolol, and Toprol may worsen it.

Since there's no good treatment, preventing HAVS is key. First, don't grip the grips tightly—it increases the risk. In general, a tight grip hurts handling. Bikes are smarter than we are. If you're going around a curve with a death grip (ahem) on the bar and hit a pothole, you're more likely to crash.

Not having to grip the throttle constantly is helpful. I've used a throttle friction screw on my BMWs for many years. It increases friction on the throttle, slowing the return. An aftermarket device called the Throttlemeister (www.throttlemeister.com) can serve the same purpose—it's also a bar-end weight. They're very well made and remarkably effective. The only problem I've found is that when using heated grips, the setting changes. Please be careful when using a throttle friction device, especially at first.

Another throttle device is the Throttle Rocker (www.throttlerocker.com), which attaches to the throttle with hook/loop fastener. It seems to work well, but I've heard of at least one rider who caught the sleeve of his riding jacket on it, causing a problem. On the other hand, it's a lot cheaper than the Throttlemeister and simpler to install.

An O-ring can provide throttle friction. A 1 x 3/16-inch rubber O-ring from the local hardware store will work, but may degrade with sunlight. Caterpillar makes O-rings in silicone and in nitrile. Silicone is softer and more UV resistant; nitrile is harder and longer lasting. Part numbers are 8M-5266 and 8B-4967 for the 24.77mm silicone and nitrile, respectively, and 8M-4991 and 5H-7370 for the 27.94mm.

Please be careful when using a throttle friction device.

Use vibration absorbers. Gloves with gel palms can help a lot. Changing your handgrips may help, too. (Hint: lubricate new grips with hairspray to slide them on easily and then have them stay in place.) Some handgrips are better than others at minimizing transmitted vibrations.

Reducing handlebar vibration will help (see tinyurl.com/QKPQW). In bikes with handlebars (as opposed to clip-ons) a bar snake (www.BarSnake.com), a device made of "non-bouncing" rubber works well. They even make a liquid Bar Snake that solidifies inside handlebars (good for tapered bars, etc.). Some folks just pour lead shot into their handlebars.

Bar end weights help. By adding mass, they decrease the resonant frequency of the bar. Heavier is better. For examples of some, go to tinyurl.com/RJ45A. Many people have told me they like the effects of Hunter's Flat-Bars, too. They're worth checking out.

In terms of specific treatment, well, there's not much available. Certain medications called "calcium channel blockers" sometimes help, but once you reach the stage of having cold, numb fingers, it may never go away entirely. In HAVS, an ounce of prevention is worth a *ton* of cure.

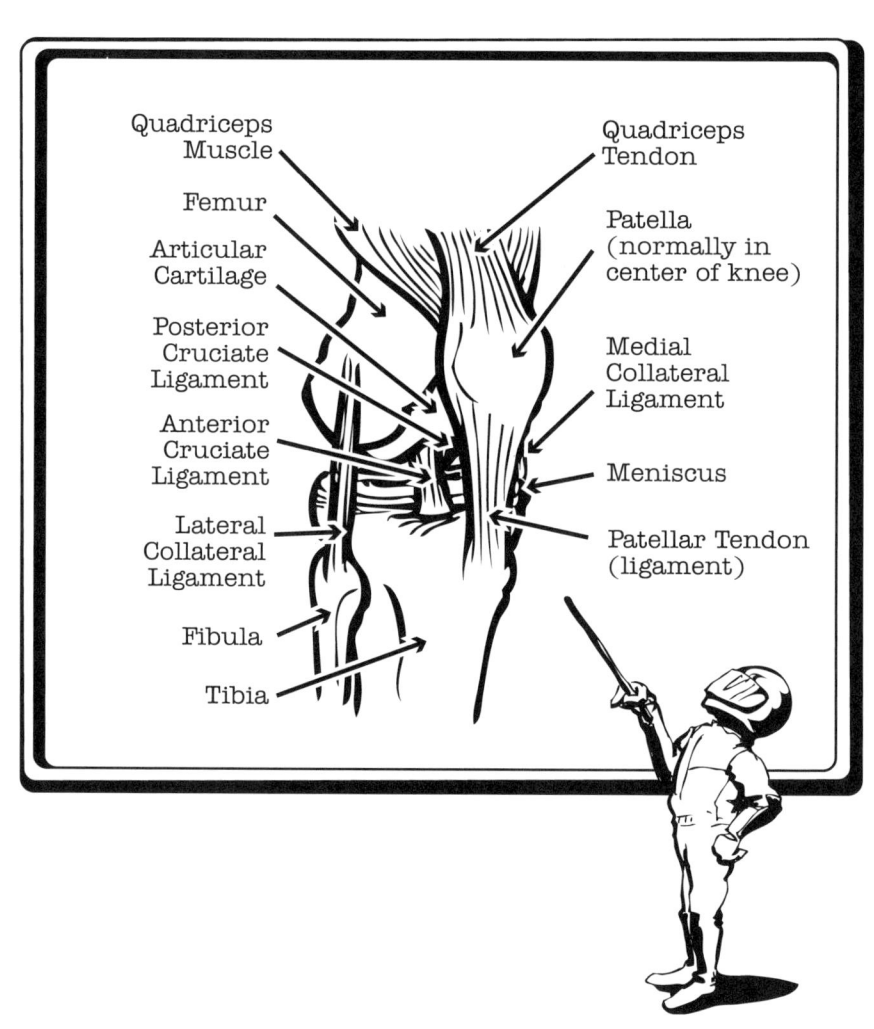

What's a Joint Like This Doing in a Nice Girl Like You?

It's a corny line, and I most often use it when I'm talking about a patient's knee. I think the knee is a bad design. If and when I meet the designer, I'll politely suggest that knees are good for quadrupeds, but unfortunately don't work well for bipeds. And don't even get me started on coronary arteries or backs! Sometimes I get the feeling that Homo Sapiens is a beta version.

The knee is one of the most commonly injured joints in motorcyclists. It's exposed to direct trauma when it hits the road, and often gets twisted during a low-side injury.

The knee's mostly a hinge joint, with the femur (thigh bone) on top and the tibia (shinbone) below. In front, the patella (kneecap) provides some protection and gives extra leverage when straightening the knee. The back of the kneecap and each end of the tibia and femur are coated with cartilage, providing padding and a slick bearing surface. There are also two pads of cartilage (the medial and lateral meniscus), which help distribute the weight of the body and the lubricating synovial fluid.

Each knee has a lateral collateral ligament along the outside and a medial collateral ligament along the inside. These help keep the knee from bending sideways. The femur and tibia are connected inside the middle of the knee joint by the anterior cruciate ligament (ACL), which prevents rotation and keeps the femur from moving backwards, and the posterior cruciate ligament (PCL), which keeps the femur from moving forward.

The quad muscles on the front of the thigh straighten the knee, as in standing from a squat. The hamstrings behind the thigh help to bend the knee against resistance.

The knee joint is the biggest joint in the body, and supports all your body's weight. Lots of things can go wrong. Some things are more common than others.

In a new knee injury, the question—Do I need to see a doctor? —often has an obvious answer. If the knee doesn't support your weight, feels unstable, gets grossly swollen, locks, or doesn't bend or straighten completely, getting it checked right away is a good idea. If it just got whacked and you can walk on it without any of the above signs, trying some RICE (rest, ice, compression, and elevation) and watching it for a couple of days isn't unreasonable.

Most significant knee injuries other than fractures involve a ligament or meniscus. They tend to act differently, though in some cases you may injure both. Ligament injuries hurt soon, usually right after the injury, but cartilages hurt slowly—often, with a cartilage tear, the knee may take hours to swell and to start hurting a lot. Even though the cartilage injury sometimes doesn't hurt as much, they're very important to diagnose. Untreated cartilage injuries may lead to arthritis by irritating the inside of the knee joint. And osteoarthritis (OA) of the knee is a very common cause of chronic knee pain and disability, as is discussed later.

Patellofemoral syndrome (PFS) is one of the most common causes of knee pain besides acute injuries. Runners get this a lot. Normally, the patella slides in a groove in the front of the femur, and is surrounded by the tendons from the four muscles on the front of the thigh, called the quadriceps muscles (or quads). These muscles mostly straighten the knee, as when you stand on your bike's pegs.

The smooth layer of cartilage on the back of the kneecap lets it slide easily over the femur. It's easy to damage this cartilage when you fall onto your knee—something we all have done. When dinged, it's very slow to heal. And when it doesn't heal right, it's not smooth, so the kneecap can scrape when it rubs over the end of the femur. In other cases of PFS, the kneecap doesn't track correctly, perhaps due to improper functioning of the muscles that act on it. PFS is most painful when the kneecap's getting pushed against the femur, like when you're standing from a crouched position, climbing stairs, spending time with your knees bent (think back seat of a compact car, or riding a sports bike), or running a lot.

Sometimes PFS flares up, especially after there's been extra wear and tear on the knees. When this happens, pushing the kneecap down against the knee while the leg is out straight, and then trying to lift the foot, really hurts. You'll sometimes feel the kneecap scrape against the femur. This is a pretty reliable indication that knee pain is due to PFS.

When PFS flares up, an NSAID like ibuprofen (Motrin, Advil) or naproxen (Aleve) can help. Icing the area (be sure to use a towel between the ice and the skin) and rest help, too. Occasionally I'll recommend a long knee splint, which keeps the knee from bending, and takes the pressure off the patella. Some physicians and therapists tape the kneecap.

Tightening the quad muscles in the front of the thigh with the leg straight (like sitting on the floor or a couch) helps, too. If PFS continues, seeing a sports medicine physician or an orthopedist is worthwhile. Sometimes very specific exercises (like vastus medialis training) may possibly improve or eliminate PFS.

Osteoarthritis of the knee is very common. Traditionally, treatment has been an NSAID like ibuprofen, naproxen (Aleve), or others. Sometimes a flare-up can be treated with a steroid injection. In the worst, most disabling cases, total knee replacement is often the cure. Some pain medications like acetaminophen (Tylenol) are safer than NSAIDs.

Recently, though, two new therapies have shown promise.

First is glucosamine sulfate as a dietary supplement. It works about as well as naproxen (though it may take months to work, rather than minutes) but has fewer side effects than an NSAID. It can be taken along with NSAIDs, too. I use it with almost every patient with OA, and often suggest using it preventively.

Injection of a hyaluronic acid product into the knee joint can help people who have failed on NSAIDs or who can't take them, and who have significant disability. Hyaluronic acid is a part of the lubricating "joint juice" inside normal knees, and both lubricates and decreases inflammation. A series of injections is given that often provides relief of pain for months to a year or so. This treatment can postpone the need for a total knee replacement for quite a while.

It's worth a shot.

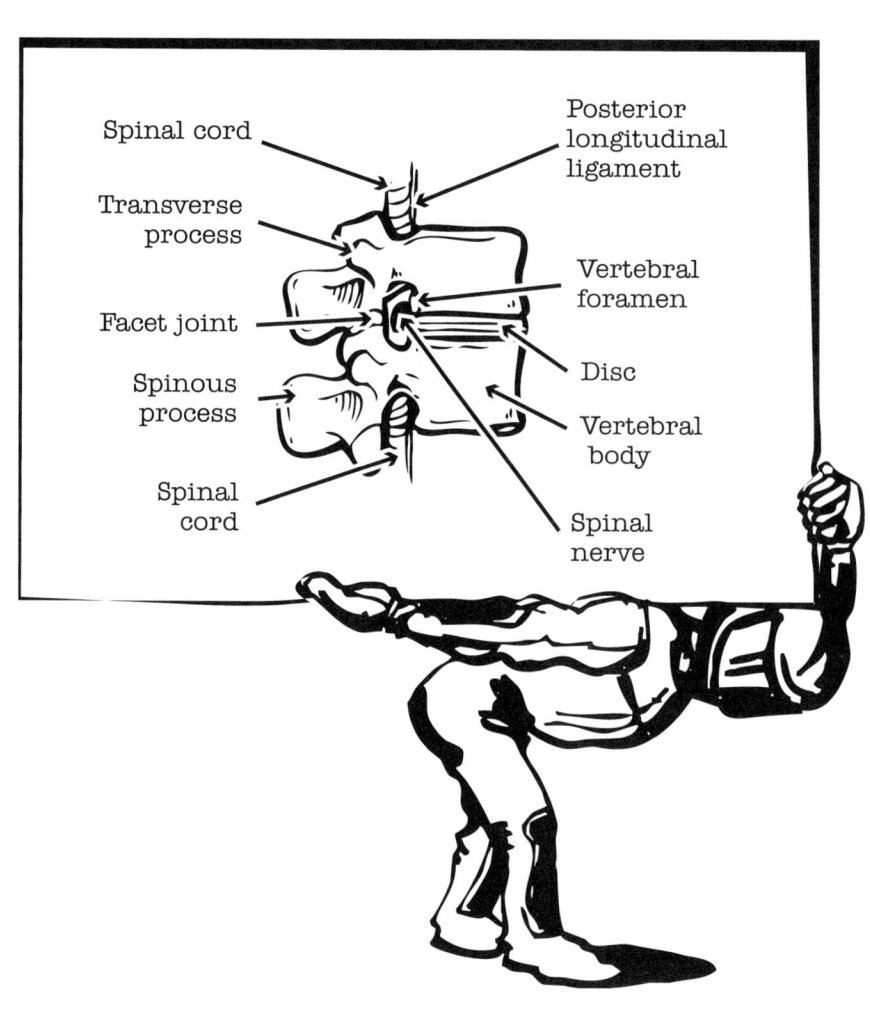

Spinal cord

Transverse process

Facet joint

Spinous process

Spinal cord

Posterior longitudinal ligament

Vertebral foramen

Disc

Vertebral body

Spinal nerve

Get Back

One day, I might meet whoever came up with the design for the human body. I hope I do. I've noticed a lot of areas needing improvement.

Knees as we have just seen are a poor design. They're ugly, easy to injure, and often wear out, requiring replacement. They're less reliable than the Lucas Electrics on old Brit bikes.

Coronary arteries are yet another problem area. How about some redundancy? At least the brain has the Circle of Willis, a ring shaped structure at the base of the brain with four inputs (two carotid and two vertebral arteries) that feeds the vessels supplying the brain. That way, the loss of one or two inputs isn't always a disaster. The heart? Nothing. One little clot and you can be a goner.

Worst of all, in my humble opinion, is the design of the back. Half of all working adults in the US have a back problem each year, of whom about one in five needs to see a professional. And back problems are the leading cause of disability in people younger than 45. Even though 90 percent of acute back problems resolve spontaneously within a month, there are plenty of problems that need specific care, such as infections, tumors, some fractures, those causing neurological deficit, and back pain due to problems in other parts of the body.

In my opinion, certain kinds of back pain are best evaluated by a medical doctor (M.D. or D.O.) as opposed to a chiropractor. These include pain that occurs immediately after an injury such as a fall or motor vehicle accident; new back pain in people under 20 or over 50; back pain with leg pain, numbness, or weakness; back pain associated with fever, vomiting, or other systemic symptoms; back pain with loss of bladder and/or bowel control; back pain that's worse while lying down, or much worse at night; pain occurring after a recent infection (like a kidney infection); or pain in people who've had cancer, or have a weakened immune system from an organ transplant, HIV, or long-term use of steroids.

On the other hand, for acute back pain that's less than a week old that doesn't fit in one of the above categories, studies show that chiropractors may do a better job than M.D.s. However, one of the best kinds of doctors for back pain is often an osteopathic physician. Their education includes most of what M.D. students get, in addition to specific training on treating back problems.

The back has several components, but the most pain nerves are in the discs, the facet joints, ligaments, and muscles attached to the back. To understand what can hurt, you need to know what the back is, and what it does.

The load bearing is done by the vertebrae, or backbones, and the discs. Each of the two dozen or so vertebrae has a cylindrical body filled with strong bone. The flexible disc is between each vertebra. The disc has a soft jelly-like inside with a tough covering called the annulus.

Behind each vertebral body is a bony arch, and inside that arch runs the spinal cord, containing the nerves connecting the body to the brain. All the arches together form the spinal canal; the top of each side of the arch touches the bottom of the arch above it, forming the "facet joint." Ligaments keep the vertebrae from moving too much (if they did, they could damage the spinal cord). There's a ligament running down the back of the vertebral bodies between them and the spinal cord, called the posterior longitudinal ligament or ligamentum flavum (yellow ligament). It's also between the spinal cord and the back of the disc.

At the top/back of each arch is a bony extension like the fin on a shark, called the spinous process, which gives back muscles a place to attach. There's a transverse process sticking out each side of the arch, too, for muscle attachment. Nerves to the body exit to the side through the space between the arches; these spaces are called the vertebral foramen.

Each pair of vertebrae forms one "spinal motion segment," which has a pair of spinal nerves exiting to the right and left, a pair of facet joints, muscles, a disc, and a pair of arches forming the spinal canal in that segment. If you understand these structures, you can understand all the many different causes of back pain. And by understanding them, you can help eliminate them by changing what you do.

For motorcyclists, a lot of what you do depends on what you ride, and the kind of riding you do. There are two extremes of riding positions. Think of a racer on a sport bike, with her back bent far forward, hips flexed, hugging the tank; and a cruiser who's leaning back, feet up on the highway pegs. These people are putting strain on different parts of their spine.

And there's more than just the riding position in terms of the effect on the back. Other equipment makes a big difference, too. If a rider has his compression damping set too high, or if his preload is off, there's going to be unnecessary repeated squeezing of the discs when he hits a pothole or a bump. This aggravates certain conditions a lot more than others.

A windscreen can make a big difference in how a ride affects your back, too. If you have a lot of wind on your torso and you have to counter that pressure with your arms and/or your abdominal muscles, you're adding to the compression forces on your back. On the other hand, if you've got a windshield that's exactly the right height, you're essentially leaning on a pillow of air, greatly reducing the load on your back. One of the nicest things about my BMW R1100RSL is the adjustable windscreen and the adjustable seat height. I can tune it to what I need.

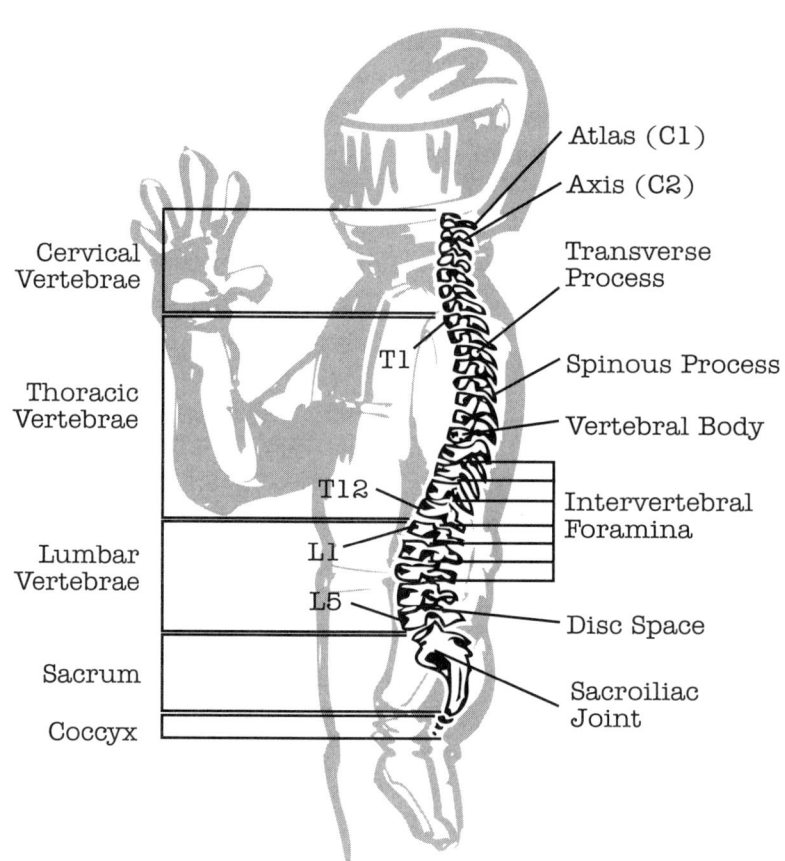

Cervical Vertebrae

Thoracic Vertebrae

Lumbar Vertebrae

Sacrum

Coccyx

T1

T12

L1

L5

Atlas (C1)

Axis (C2)

Transverse Process

Spinous Process

Vertebral Body

Intervertebral Foramina

Disc Space

Sacroiliac Joint

Backs Gone Bad

This may seem counterintuitive, but the stomach is one of the most important parts of the back. Use the illustration to imagine, if you will, looking at a skeleton from the side. The skeleton is facing to the left, and the back makes a gentle S-shaped curve. Below the neck (the cervical vertebrae) the thoracic vertebrae curve to the left over the shoulders and the lumbar vertebrae curve the other way behind the abdomen.

The bottom of the spine is attached to the back of the ring of the pelvis, which is roughly horizontal. If you push your stomach out, you increase the curvature behind your abdomen (increasing the "lordotic" curve) by tilting the front of the pelvis downward. To pull your stomach in, you pull up the front of your pelvis using your abdominal muscles, flattening the lordotic curve of your lower lumbar spine.

Think of the soft discs between your lumbar vertebrae. If your lumbar spine is curved a lot (i.e., if your stomach is hanging out) the backs of the vertebrae are closer together, squeezing the back of the lumbar discs. When you're bent forward, there's a lot less curvature, and there's more pressure on the front of the discs. Weak stomach muscles can really hurt a bad back.

When your stomach muscles are strong, they pull up the front of your pelvis all the time. This reduces excessive lordotic curve, and helps relieve squeezing of the discs. Be careful when doing stomach exercises, though—sit-ups can hurt your back. Crunches, when done correctly (keeping your neck straight) can be safer.

Sadly, lumbar discs don't last. Half of the people over 50 have dried out or protruding discs. Remember how nerves exit between the arches (the foramina) on each side of the spine? When bulging, discs may push on the nerve—this is called a radiculopathy. If it's your leg, it's called "sciatica."

Common wisdom once was that discs affected nerves mostly by direct pressure; now it seems that back pain can be caused by the fluids inside the disc leaking out and irritating the nerve. It follows that decreasing fluid leakage lessens pain.

Think again of the spinal motion segment, composed of a disc and two vertebrae, one above and one below. Forward bending squeezes the disc, causing it to leak irritating disc fluid. Back bending can decrease the opening between the arches on each side (the foramina), directly irritating nerve roots.

Picture someone crouched over a race bike. Her back is bent forward, squeezing the front of the discs—there's no lordotic curve at all. If she's got a leaky disc, it'll ooze irritating disc juice onto the nerve roots, causing pain and inflammation.

Imagine a cruiser rider, leaning back, legs out. His lumbar spine isn't bent forward—it's probably bent back, especially if the rider's gut pushes the front of the pelvis down. Without a screen, wind pressure on the chest has to be countered by stomach muscles or arms, causing low back compression. This can also cause discs to leak. Windscreens can be a tremendous help for bad backs.

Remember the facet joints? They join each side of the arch behind the vertebrae to the one above and below it. Like all joints, they get arthritis (i.e., "joint inflammation"). Arthritic joints swell, and arthritic facet joints put pressure on nerve roots passing through the foramina.

To diagnose facet arthritis, I have patients sit backwards on a chair (or on a non-revolving stool). I pull their shoulders back about a foot; then a foot to the side, and then straight forward. This maneuver grinds the facet joints on that side of the lumbar spine—doing it toward the other side grinds the opposite ones. If the facet joint is bad, this causes pain. If a patient has this problem, a windscreen and/or more forward bars helps to unload the facet joints.

Excess body weight is bad for backs. Many of us weigh more as we age. Gaining 40 pounds since age 20 isn't uncommon. If this is true for you, next time you're at Costco or Sam's Club, pick up a full 5-gallon container and carry it around a while, if you can. Your back carries this much extra weight around all day. No wonder it hurts.

Treatment for back problems depends on what the problem is. Sciatica, for example, is due to a nerve being affected by pressure or irritating disc juice. In most cases, anti-inflammatory medications help. Though ibuprofen (Advil/Nuprin/Motrin) is fast and effective, it only lasts 4 hours or so. I've had better luck with long-lasting NSAIDs like naproxen (Aleve) taken three times a day with meals. Folks with a sensitive stomach may tolerate these kind of medications better with an acid-reducer like omeprazole (available without prescription as Prilosec OTC) taken a half hour before breakfast every day.

Physical therapy is very good for back complaints, too. A good therapist can pinpoint problems like excess curvature due to abdominal muscle weakness and give you an appropriate home exercise program. Your doctor can recommend a good therapist and prescribe therapy.

Cortisone injections into a swollen, inflamed facet joint, or around swollen irritated nerve roots are sometimes very useful, especially if NSAIDs and PT aren't enough. These injections are done by orthopedists, radiologists, and sometimes physiatrists (physical medicine & rehabilitation experts).

Surgery is the last resort for back problems, although newer procedures like mini-discectomy don't have the longer down time associated with laminectomy. There are minimally-invasive ways to help disc problems, too, that may be worth considering.

In general, surgery's indicated for progressive nerve problems (weakness, numbness) or uncontrollable pain—and it's generally most helpful for cases with a lot of pain in the leg, not the back.

And last, a good saddle can really help your back, in my experience. Mine's an old Bill Mayer (Senior). That, and my BMW R1100RS's adjustable windshield, seat height, and clip-on hand grips, have allowed me to ride 14 hour days without any back pain at all!

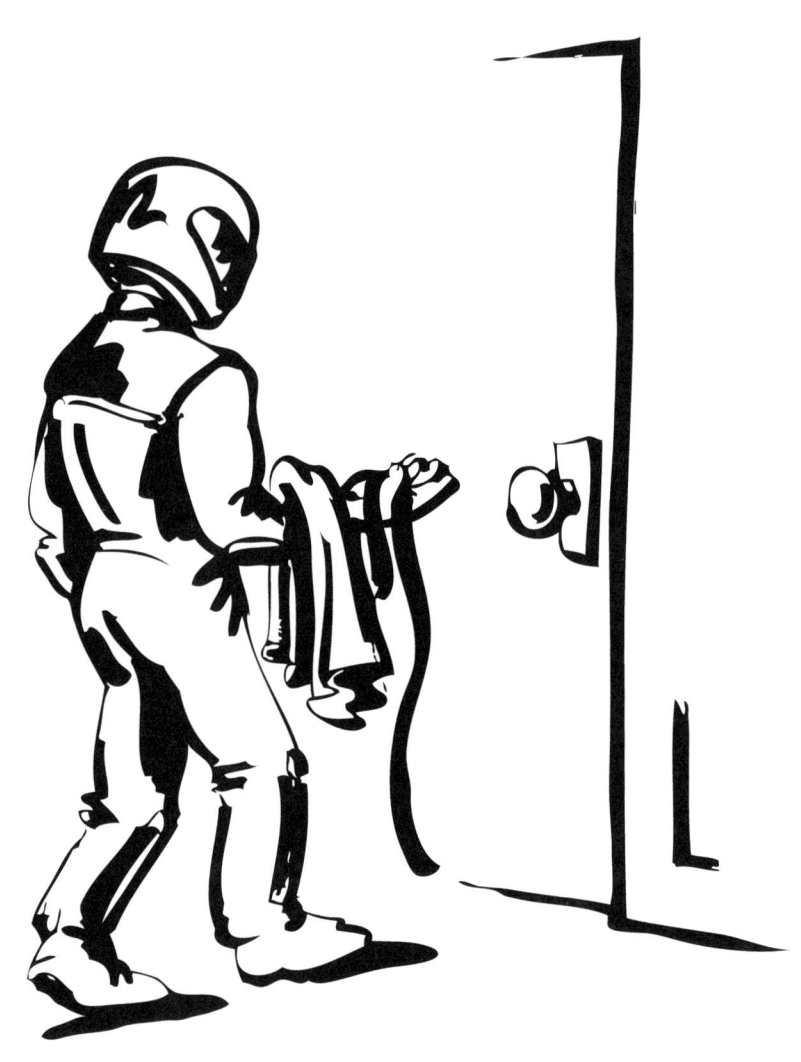

A Pain in the Neck

Lots of folks have a pinched nerve in their neck (a cervical radiculopathy) and don't know it. Pain in the shoulder or arm that you can make worse by tilting or turning your head is probably due to a pinched nerve, even without neck pain.

The neck has seven bones (vertebrae). Each has a solid round body with an arch behind it (the posterior elements). These posterior elements have joints (called "facet joints") that keep the vertebrae in line. Your spinal cord is inside the arch, within the spinal canal. The "foramen" on each side are where nerves to your neck, shoulders, and arms come out. Between each vertebral body is a soft disc, providing padding and helping the neck bend and turn. These have a tough covering with a soft inside. Think of a jelly donut.

There are several things that can pinch nerves. The inside part of a disc may push through its covering (a ruptured or herniated disc) or a disc may bulge, pushing on the nerve as it leaves the spinal cord. Nerve pressure can cause pain, tingling, weakness, numbness, or paralysis. Mild pressure that only produces pain on and off is more likely to get better by itself, since a ruptured disc often dries up and shrinks over several months' time. I've even known cases that have had constant pain and significant weakness in the arm to get better without surgery. But with these symptoms, you should seek medical care. And if you develop these symptoms after an injury—see a physician before trying any of these suggestions.

In some cases, the nerve gets pinched as it comes through the foramen between two vertebrae. Sometimes there are "bone spurs" in this area that can irritate or push on the nerve. Arthritis in the facet joints may also do this. Muscle spasms may squeeze a nerve tightly enough to produce some of the symptoms mentioned above. Usually, though, the spasm only produces pain or tingling—paralysis and/or total numbness is unusual.

Pain is an early symptom of nerve pressure. Sometimes pain is constant, at other times it comes after work or after standing, sitting, walking, or riding. It sometimes feels like an ache or a burning—some folks say it feels like "ice water." Tingling is also common with a pinched nerve, and may indicate there's more pressure on the nerve than only pain indicates. Numbness and weakness/paralysis are more serious symptoms. If your arm is numb—that is, if it feels like your lip does after you visit the dentist, and you can pinch it or stick it with something sharp and not feel it—you must seek care promptly. Nerve pressure causing numbness must be treated before it damages the nerve permanently. Weakness or paralysis is another symptom. If you've lost strength in your hand, arm, or shoulder, and have symptoms of a pinched nerve, get it checked without delay, even if it doesn't hurt. Other conditions, like strokes or stroke warnings, can produce these symptoms, too.

On a bike, there are several things you can do that may help if you've got a pinched nerve. Bar-backs that raise the handlebars and move them backwards can be helpful, especially on sportbikes. Different handlebars can do the same. Often, a windshield changes the wind pressure on your head, which changes how your neck muscles are working as you ride. Depending on your individual problem, your bike, your height, etc., you may do better with or without a windshield. Experiment.

You can try treating a mild cervical radiculopathy yourself. Medicines, like Advil, Nuprin, Motrin (ibuprofen), or Aleve (naproxen) are helpful. I often recommend up to 2400 mg of ibuprofen a day in divided doses, but only with food. *Not* compressing the spine by bouncing along a dirt road, or by jumping down from a height (even as little as a foot or two) helps.

IMPORTANT NOTE: If you have neck pain or any of these symptoms after an accident, or after a head or neck injury, see a physician before trying home traction.

Home traction is one of the most helpful treatments in my experience—I've used it on myself for years. All you need is a small towel or laundry bag, a piece of rope or cord, and a doorknob. First, tie one end of the cord to one end of the towel. Then loop it over the doorknob, bring it back and tie it to other end of the towel. You want it to be just long enough that the middle of the towel barely touches the floor when hanging from the doorknob.

Next, lie down on your back with the top of your head close to the door. Rest the back of your head from your ears down in the sling formed by the towel. Your head should be held comfortably, just barely off the floor—it should not be tilted forward or back. If you do this correctly, it should be pretty comfortable. It's helpful to wiggle your head side-to-side a little bit now and then while you're lying there. It should feel comfortable. If it hurts, or makes your neck, arm, or shoulder feel worse, *don't do it.*

Lie there for only seven minutes on the first day. It might feel good right away, or you might not feel any difference. But, doing it for too long may stretch your neck muscles and make them cramp, and you'll feel worse. You can do it twice the first day if you like, at least eight hours apart. Then add one minute a day until you get to 15 minutes, twice daily. Continue at 15 minutes twice a day for as long as you need to, depending on symptoms. This may relieve the pressure on the nerve, allowing it to recover. With less irritation, swelling often decreases, so it's not pinched anymore. Most folks feel a little better after the first day or so, and the benefit increases daily.

A couple of pointers: Make sure you have a loud timer with you, so you don't fall asleep. If you do, you may overstretch your neck muscles, which may make them cramp, worsening the problem. Also (this is very important), be sure to lock the door so nobody comes through it while you're lying there.

Don't ask me how I know this.

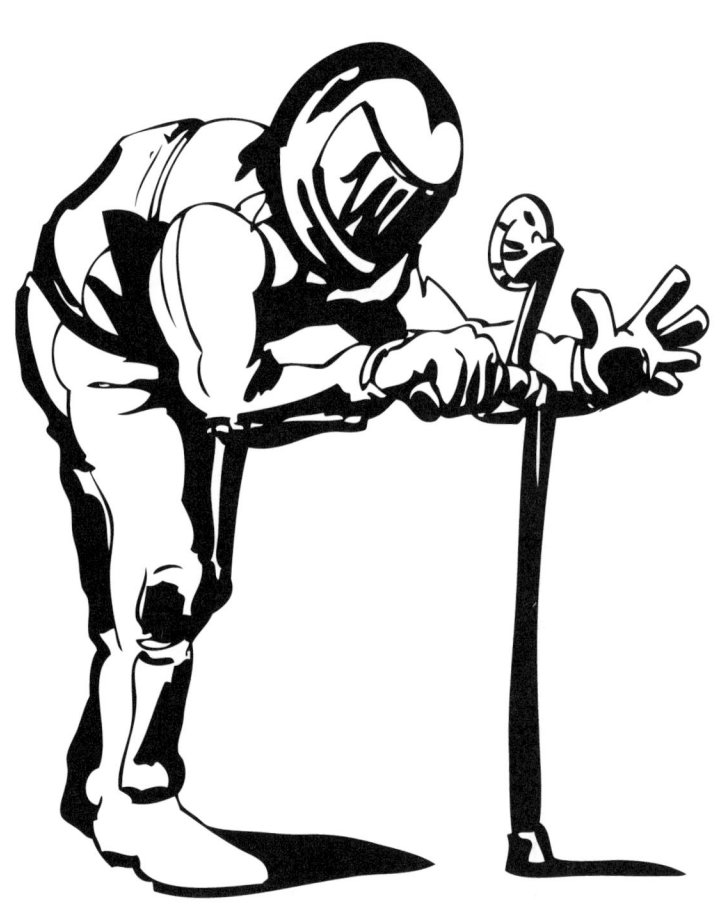

These Old Bones

I'm often asked, "Is it safe to keep riding when I get old?" That's a logical question, considering some of the normal changes the body goes through. Understanding these changes is useful. It's knowing the territory ahead. Since those of us who are lucky will get old, consider this a roadmap into aging.

Aging causes stiffer joints and more brittle bones. Our joints age from loss of cartilage, which provides both lubrication and padding. Actual arthritis (most commonly, osteoarthritis) affects one in seven Americans, causing more disability than back pain, heart or lung conditions, diabetes, or cancer. It affects 60 percent of men and 70 percent of women over 65. The knees are most commonly involved in osteoarthritis.

Osteoarthritis is linked to joint trauma, which can be acute (like a fracture), intermittent (like recurrent dislocations, commonly at the shoulder), or repetitive (being overweight). Other kinds of arthritis can occur. Rheumatoid arthritis, for example, is due to the body attacking itself with its own immune system.

There are a number of treatments for osteoarthritis. NSAIDs like aspirin, ibuprofen, and naproxen are commonly used, and help with pain and inflammation. However, they're hazardous to your stomach, especially if you smoke, drink, take steroids (like prednisone) or have an ulcer history. Expensive, prescription-only cox-2 inhibitors like Celebrex® lower the risk, as does omeprazole (Prilosec OTC®) which is available without prescription. The danger of NSAIDs is substantial, especially as you get older. Taking them increases the risk of bleeding or ulcer about four times, and they can cause damage even without causing any stomach upset or discomfort. Each year, about 50,000 people are hospitalized and almost 4,000 die from taking these medications. That's as many deaths as there are from motorcycle accidents. Painkillers like acetaminophen (Tylenol®) are safe, effective, and often underused.

Glucosamine sulfate, taken every day as a supplement, may help treat and prevent osteoarthritis by slowing the normal loss of cartilage. It may take six months or more to make a difference, though. Glucosamine has no side effects, unlike NSAIDs. Many good studies have shown it to be about as effective as naproxen for knee osteoarthritis.

Another helpful treatment is viscosupplementation, which involves a series of three injections of "artificial joint fluid," which was first used on knees. Joints with osteoarthritis tend to have low levels of healthy joint fluid. Think of viscosupplementation as a "lube job" which sometimes provides many months of pain relief. Although it can't be used in people with egg allergies, and occasionally causes some local discomfort, I've seen some remarkably good results.

Another technique in osteoarthritis treatment is grafting of cartilage, either an allograft from a dead donor, or from another part of your own body (an autograft). This is usually reserved for younger patients—once the joint's got advanced arthritis, it's unlikely to work as well. For more info on this or viscosupplementation, see an orthopedist, especially one with an interest in sports medicine.

It doesn't help to have good joints if your bones are weak. As we get more sedentary, our bones get weaker. This is because bones automatically get stronger when they're subjected to a more weight-bearing load, and weaken if they're not used. If we sit on our duff all day, bones slowly lose calcium and strength. This eventually can lead to osteopenia and osteoporosis.

You can think of osteopenia as "thinning bones" and osteoporosis as "porous bones." Osteoporosis is worse. It greatly increases the risk of fracture. Not only that, it's all too common. Half of all women and an eighth of all men in the U.S. will have a fracture due to osteoporosis in their lifetime. Each year there are about 800,000 spine fractures, 300,000 hip fractures, and 250,000 wrist fractures from osteoporosis in the U.S. Some prescription medications may stop or reverse it.

It's easy to check for osteoporosis with a "bone mineral density" test. (tinyurl.com/7NCSR). Typically, these are done on postmenopausal women at higher risk for fractures. However, men are at risk too, especially as they get older. Long-term steroid use greatly increases risk, as does significant weight loss.

The spine fractures can occur for little or no reason. I had an elderly patient who broke her back while lifting some laundry from her washing machine. Not only do fractured spines cause a lot of pain, they lead to more fractures. Here's how:

When a vertebra in the spine fractures from osteoporosis, it's typically what's called a compression fracture, in which the front of the vertebra collapses, resulting in what's called a wedge deformity. This tilts the spine and the rest of the body above the fracture forward. Unfortunately, this forward tilt puts more pressure on the front part of the vertebrae around the broken one, making them more likely to fracture, too. The end result of these fractures is the bent-forward posture you sometimes see in older women—it's sometimes called the "dowager's hump."

The bent-forward posture puts pressure on the lungs and abdominal organs, which makes it important to relieve the pressure. Dr. Mark Reily invented a very interesting procedure called a "balloon kyphoplasty," in which a balloon is inserted into the collapsed vertebra, and then inflated to reverse the wedging (see

Balloon Kyphoplasty

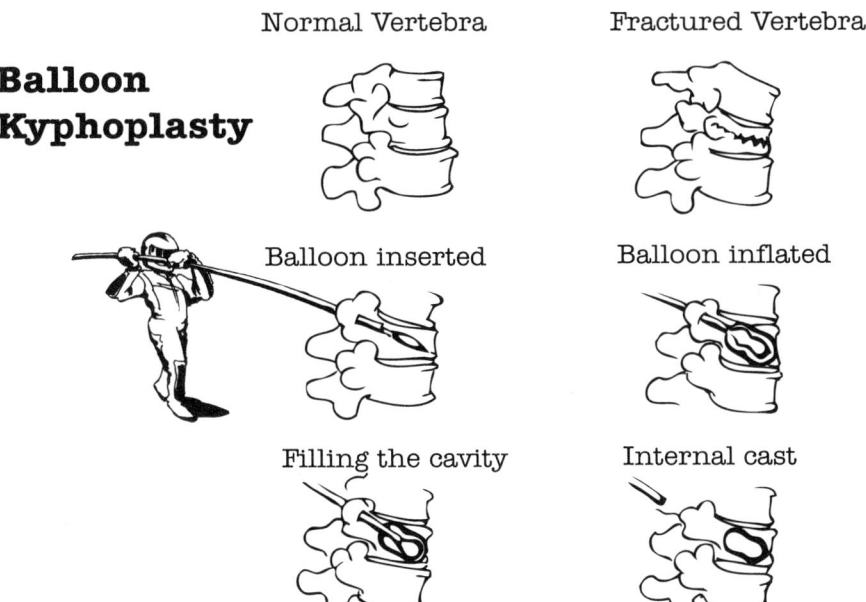

Normal Vertebra

Fractured Vertebra

Balloon inserted

Balloon inflated

Filling the cavity

Internal cast

tinyurl.com/78XF3). Bone cement is then injected into the hollow spaces made by the balloon, which maintains the vertebra's restored normal shape. It doesn't work in healthy bone that's fractured in an injury, though—but in softer, osteoporotic bone it can help tremendously, as it can in bone eaten away by cancer (like metastatic prostate, lung, or breast cancer, or in myeloma).

Preventing osteoporosis is a good idea for motorcyclists, since we're occasionally in situations where weaker bones get broken. Be sure to get 1500 to 2000 mg of USP calcium daily (the USP on the label means "no lead or bad stuff"). Get at least 20 times your age in vitamin D daily, too. And if you've got osteoporosis, be sure to include 1000 units of vitamin D daily with the medications your doctor prescribed.

Remember: The bones you save can be your own.

Don't Blink!

Your cornea (the clear part of your eye) is the most sensitive part of your body. If you doubt that, try not blinking for 60 seconds. Most folks have trouble keeping their eyes open that long—the slight drying you get in that time causes enough discomfort that blinking becomes involuntary.

If air can cause discomfort to your cornea, a piece of road grit can be much worse. We've all gotten something in our eye (called a "corneal foreign body") at times, and getting rid of it immediately becomes our top priority. Like most things, there's a right and a wrong way to do this.

Never try to use anything like a tissue, Q-tip, cloth, or a wet fingertip to remove something that's on the cornea. Though that's okay for an eyelash that's in the sack under the eye, away from the clear part, the cornea is very soft and extremely easy to damage. I see patients all the time who tried wiping out a bit of grit with a tissue and ended up wiping away a big piece of the surface of the cornea. This hurts a lot, and takes days to heal.

Leaving the grit until you can get to a doctor or ER is safer, but gives it time to sink into the soft surface of the cornea, which means the doc has to dig it out with a needle or other instrument. Metallic foreign bodies can even start rusting, leaving you with a small tattoo called a "rust ring" that needs to be removed. If you can remove it safely and quickly you're way ahead of the game. And by quickly, I mean stopping what you're doing and taking it out right then. Don't wait 10 minutes until you get home, or it's more likely to start digging into your cornea.

The only thing that's safe to use on your cornea is the inside of your eyelid. Here's a technique that's almost always been successful in my experience.

Grab your eyelashes and pull the upper lid forward, away from your eyeball. While holding it away from the eye, look UP as high as possible. Then pull the eyelid down as far as it will comfortably

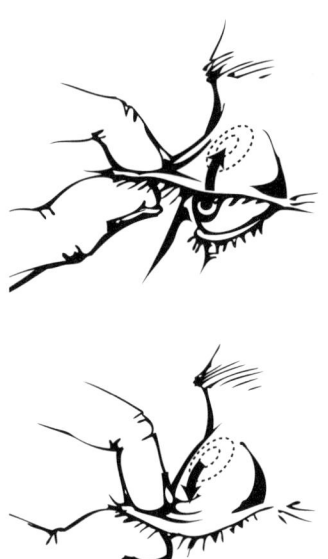

go, laying it against the lower eyelid. While holding it there, look DOWN so your eyeball rotates downward. Release the eyelashes, and blink a few times. That should do the trick. If it's not better, just repeat.

Though a corneal foreign body is painful, it's not particularly dangerous. A foreign body that penetrates the eye can be very dangerous, and sometimes isn't as painful as something on the cornea. This can happen when you're working with metal, and a piece of it hits your eye at high speed. A metal-on-metal impact like when you hit metal with a hammer is the usual cause.

Sometimes you'll just feel a little pain in the eye that then gets better for a while. Sometimes you might not feel much at all, depending on where the eye was penetrated. If you get a foreign body that penetrates the eyeball, and it's not promptly removed (and sometimes even if it is), that eye may go blind. What's even worse, this can set up a process where your body then rejects your remaining good eye, and it goes blind, too. Remember, this only happens if a piece of metal is driven *inside* your eyeball—not the typical situation. That's why eye protection is so important. If you don't have good safety goggles, just wear your helmet with the visor down when using a grinder or other hazardous equipment.

Another painful eye problem is something caught on the inside of your eyelid. This scratches your eyeball every time you blink, and it hurts a lot. This is pretty easy to treat—all you need to do is turn the eyelid inside out to look under it. Of course, this is best done with the help of another person—it's tough to do on yourself.

First, take something small and dull, like a Q-tip, the tip of a pen or pencil, or a key, and put it against the top part of the eyelid. Then ask the patient to look down, and fold the lid back over the pencil tip. There's a semi-rigid plate made out of cartilage in the bottom half of the eyelid that can be flipped over the pencil or Q-tip. The lid then will stay up and let you inspect the bottom of the upper lid, preferably with good light and magnification. If there's something there, you can wipe it away with a Q-tip or the wet corner of a tissue. This part of the eye isn't as delicate as the cornea, which you should never touch with anything.

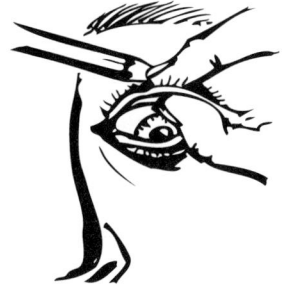

If you think you've scraped your cornea, get it checked. The doc will numb up the eye with a local anesthetic, and then examine it with fluorescein, which shows any area of the cornea that's been damaged. You'll probably get a prescription for an antibiotic eye drop, and depending on the damage, the doc might

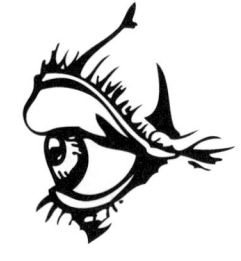

want to patch the eye, and will sometimes put in a drop that paralyzes the iris, which then dilates your pupil. This helps prevent the iris from cramping, causing pain. If she does dilate your eye, remember that you'll need sunglasses for a day or so.

Most corneal scrapes and superficial injuries heal in one or two days. Usually, an over-the-counter medicine like Advil, Nuprin, or Aleve is enough for the pain of a minor scrape. If the pain was considerable, ask the doc if she thinks you need anything stronger than that. Last—don't even *think* of riding your bike home if your eye was patched. You'll have impaired depth perception and might end up right back in the hospital.

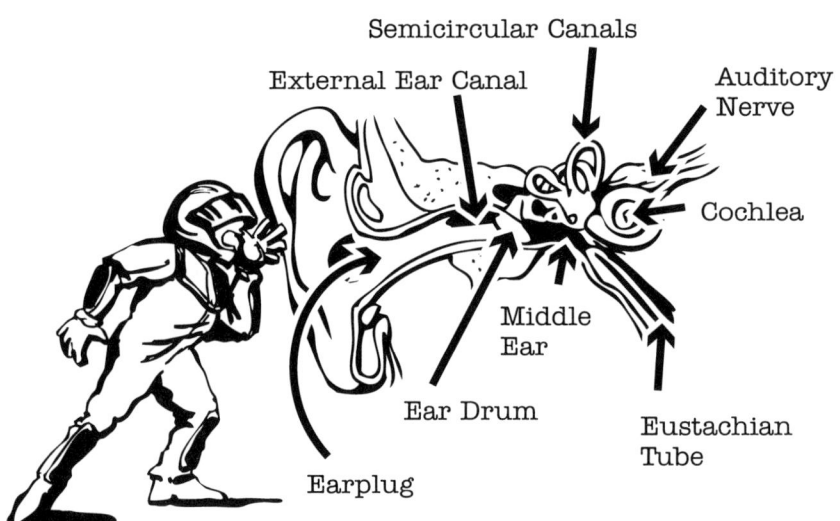

Semicircular Canals

External Ear Canal

Auditory Nerve

Cochlea

Middle Ear

Ear Drum

Eustachian Tube

Earplug

Earplugs

Are earplugs good or bad? Some say "earplugs muffle warning sounds like horns, sirens, and other dangers." But others say, "if I don't wear earplugs while riding, I'll lose my hearing." Who's right?

I've got a strong bias on this subject—I'm a big proponent of hearing protection. Back in the 1980s, I started "H.E.A.R.," (www.Hearnet.com). I believe all riders benefit from earplugs when riding at highway speeds.

Ears evolved to be sensitive to the faintest sounds. The mammal that heard the predator creeping up on it had an evolutionary advantage. Consequently, the ear evolved into an incredibly sensitive organ. The outer ear, or pinna, gives directionality to sounds. It also helps "scoop up" sound waves and channels them down the ear canal. When we cup a hand behind our ears, we amplify this effect.

The ear canal amplifies sound by a factor of 10 or more before it gets to the end of the canal, hitting the eardrum. It's a flexible membrane, like a drumhead, and moves when sound waves hit it. When the eardrum moves, the tiny bone attached to its inside, called the hammer or "malleus," moves, too. This moves the anvil, or "incus," which in turn moves the stirrup or "stapes," that's connected to a tiny window in the hearing organ, "cochlea" that contains the hair cells that actually do the hearing. In the cochlea, the vibrations stimulate tiny hair cells, which vibrate at different frequencies. They then send signals to the auditory center of the brain, which interprets them.

The canal amplifies sounds by a factor of 10. The eardrum is 15 to 30 times the size of the window in the cochlea, so it amplifies by a factor of 15 to 30. The bones triple the sound levels, due to leverage. Overall, the sounds getting to your inner ear have been mechanically amplified by a factor of up to 900—almost 1000 times louder. The ear's an incredibly sensitive organ. Sometimes, it's too sensitive.

To temporarily reduce sensitivity, we have the stapedius muscle in the middle ear, attached to the stapes. Loud sounds make it contract, muffling the noise. It also contracts before speaking or chewing, protecting us against our own sounds.

But continuous loud sounds are unnatural. The auditory system evolved to pick up quiet sounds, like the saber-tooth tiger sneaking up on you. There were no continuous loud sounds when ears evolved. Could it be that we hear better with less sound coming in?

It's been proven that earplugs improve the ability of riders to hear sirens, horns, etc., at highway speeds, probably due to lowering volumes to a level where our auditory systems are most sensitive. Not only do earplugs improve hearing at highway speeds, they prevent hearing damage. Riding without earplugs exposes our ears to about 110 decibels. Just fifteen minutes of this gives us a day's maximum permitted noise exposure. More than that can cause permanent changes in hearing.

A phenomenon called the "temporary threshold shift," or TTS, can result from noise exposure loud enough to permanently damage hearing. Here's how you can check yourself for a TTS.

Before the sound exposure, turn a radio to an all-talk station while in a quiet room (or in your car, with the engine off and windows shut). Lower the volume until you can just barely understand all the words. This is your "hearing threshold." Leave the volume where it is.

Immediately after the noise exposure, see if you can still understand everything as well as you could before, at the same volume. If you can't, you've suffered a temporary threshold shift, which tells you the sound levels have been high enough to produce permanent hearing loss with time.

To prevent hearing loss in these situations, you can rest your ears several times an hour. This lets your hair cells "catch their breath," preventing them from dying and causing permanent loss.

It's much easier, though, to just wear earplugs. When inserted properly, good earplugs lower sound levels to a safe range. I've used both disposable foam plugs and custom-made plugs myself. The custom plugs can be used for years, and when made by someone who knows about motorcycling and helmets, provide excellent protection. They're easier than foam plugs to put in correctly, and when made right, are very comfortable. My problem is that I keep losing them.

Foam plugs can be just as effective at cutting sound levels, but putting them in correctly takes some practice. First, roll the plug back and forth between your thumb and index finger to make a skinny cylinder. Then, pull the ear back with the opposite hand behind your head while inserting the plug deeply into the ear canal. Hold it in as the plug expands, thus muffling sounds. I like foam plugs with a cord attached, making them much easier to remove and carry, and I reuse foam plugs for weeks. I've practiced enough that I can put both plugs in simultaneously—I'd be happy to show you how, in person. Just ask. I always carry earplugs.

You can tell if you've inserted a foam plug correctly by looking at its shape right after you remove it. There should be a noticeable "S" curve. If you don't see it, you probably didn't put it in deeply enough.

Earplugs provide another specific advantage to motorcyclists—they help you relax while riding. When things are quiet and peaceful, you don't get as tired during a ride. It's much easier to enjoy a ride, and to ride more safely, if you're relaxed. The Iron Butt Association Archive of Wisdom says, "Eliminate all distractions and potential irritants," and earplugs help meet that goal. David Hough writes, "It's very important to wear your earplugs," in his excellent book, *Proficient Motorcycling*.

Here's the bottom line—wearing earplugs helps you:
• Hear warning sounds better
• Save your hearing
• Enjoy your ride
• Arrive more relaxed

But, if you want to be unsafe, hearing impaired, uncomfortable, and tense, don't wear earplugs. But be prepared to wear hearing aids later.

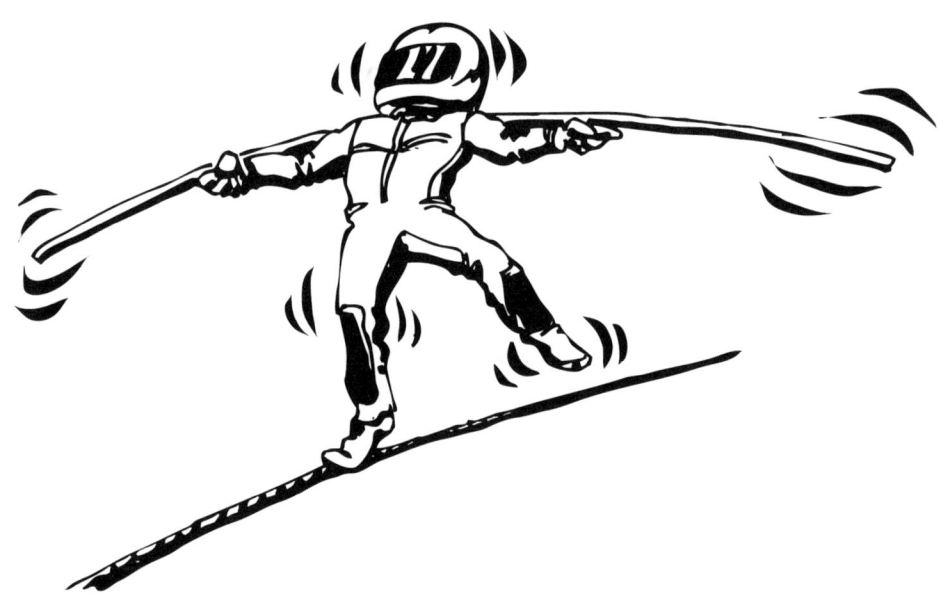

The Balancing Act

Walking on our hind legs (and riding on two wheels) requires balance. Balance involves vision, muscle/tendon sense, pressure sensors in the skin, as well as the balance sensing organ (the labyrinth) in your inner ear.

Different conditions can affect our sense of balance, including problems with the balance organ, problems in the brain itself, systemic health problems, and problems with blood flow. The most common ones are those affecting the labyrinth, including Benign Positional Vertigo (BPV), MéniPre's disease, labyrinthitis, vestibular neuronitis, and perilymph fistula.

One of the most common causes of dizziness is associated with head motion. Benign Positional Vertigo (BPV). I've suffered from this myself, and it can make riding a bike, *umm,* very interesting. Luckily, it can often be fixed.

Another common cause of balance loss, which is of more interest to us motorcyclists, is post-traumatic vertigo. (Note: Sometimes, this is caused by an inner-ear fluid leak—a perilymph fistula. Techniques described here won't work for this). After getting hit on the head, some people develop balance problems. I had a patient who'd rolled his pickup driving to the Burning Man Festival. Months later, he could only balance by holding on to the wall while walking. When he left my office half an hour later, he was cured. Here's how:

The labyrinth (balance organ) has two parts—the semicircular canals and the otolith organs (the saccule and the utricle). The semicircular canals sense rotation, and the saccule and utricle sense vertical and horizontal acceleration respectively. Both use sensitive hair cells, and both are filled with a fluid called endolymph.

There are three semicircular canals in each inner ear. The canals are ring-shaped, and have a collection of hair cells in a swelling called the ampulla that sense motion as the fluid moves past them. Obviously, fluid moves at a different speed depending on the direction of head motion relative to the plane of the canal. Since each of the three semicircular canals in each inner ear is at right angles to each other, they can sense pitch, roll, and yaw. And since the right and left balance organs are at right angles, they're very sensitive in detecting all head motions.

The otolith organs, the saccule and utricle, have flat plates of gelatinous material with small, dense calcium deposits called otoliths (Latin for "ear rocks") attached. When your head moves upward and downward (like in an elevator) the layer in the saccule moves; when you accelerate or decelerate, the layer in the utricle moves. These organs are also sensitive to head position, since tilting the head will cause the rocks to pull in a different direction. (Yes, we've actually got rocks in our heads).

In benign positional vertigo (BPV) one of the rocks gets loose and ends up in one of the semicircular canals. Some cases of posttraumatic vertigo happen for the same reason. Typically, the rock will end up in the posterior canal, since it's the lowest one, hanging down like the trap in the drain under your kitchen sink. When there's a loose rock there, it affects the flow of fluid in that semicircular canal which causes dizziness with head motions, some more than others.

In BPV, head motion/turning causes dizziness; typically, turning over in bed, looking upward quickly (in fact, BPV is also called "Top-Shelf Vertigo,"), and especially lying down or sitting up with the head turned to one side. When we do this maneuver in the office, it's called a "Dix-Hallpike Test" and says whether you've got a loose rock and which inner ear is affected.

Here's how to do a Dix-Hallpike. Put a pillow on the middle of the bed so it's under your shoulders and your head hangs back at a 45° angle when you're lying down. Sit up in bed, turn your head 45° to the right, and while keeping your head turned to the right, lie down quickly. Your head should stop tilted 45° back and turned 45° to the *right*.

If this produces *lots* of dizziness and is associated with twitching of your eyes (have a friend watch) then the *right* posterior canal is probably where the rock is. If you get so dizzy you throw up (which is not very common but does happen sometimes) that's a pretty good sign you've located the problem. If so, here's how to fix

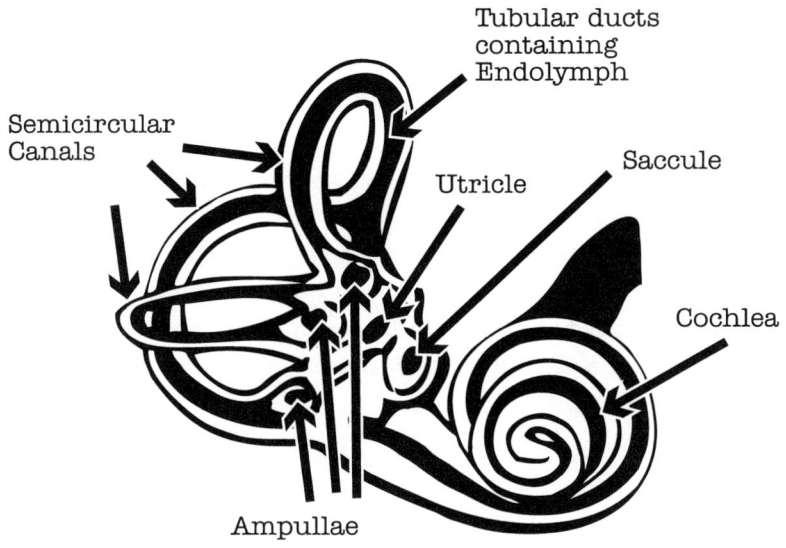

Semicircular Canals

Tubular ducts containing Endolymph

Utricle

Saccule

Cochlea

Ampullae

it. Note: Though this usually works, there are no guarantees. It's possible the dizziness might worsen, and it can cause nausea. Note that these instructions are for a loose rock in the *right* inner ear—they should be reversed for a rock on the *left*.

After lying back and getting the dizziness, keep your head tilted in the same direction for 30 to 60 seconds until the dizziness subsides. Then turn your head 90° to the left, still tilted back. Again, wait until the dizziness is gone, then turn your head and body another 135° left so you're looking straight down toward the floor. Hold until the dizziness stops, and then slowly sit up. Chances are pretty good that this will have rolled the otolith (ear rock) into an area where it won't cause dizziness. An illustration of this technique can be seen at tinyurl.com/6MVSE. (Note: I only recommend the Modified Epley Maneuver.)

After doing this, you should not lie flat on your back for 48 hours. It's best to sleep in a recliner or propped up on pillows. Also, for a week, it's a good idea not to bend over all the way. Think of the rock as if it's sitting in a tumbler glued to the top of your head. Don't let it tip out. After a week it'll probably get stuck where it is, and won't cause problems.

If this doesn't work, it can be repeated a few times a day until better. This technique can cure over 90 percent of the cases of BPV.

One point: On occasion, the dizziness caused by this technique can cause nausea and even vomiting. Keep a barf bucket, paper towel, and a glass of water handy, just in case. And of course, *don't* do this right after an accident to a rider who's dizzy. It's important to be sure there are no other injuries, like a neck fracture. But if you or a friend's been having head-motion dizziness for months to years, this might be the answer. And if you don't feel comfortable trying this, ask your family doctor, an audiologist, a neurologist, or an ear, nose and throat doc if they can help.

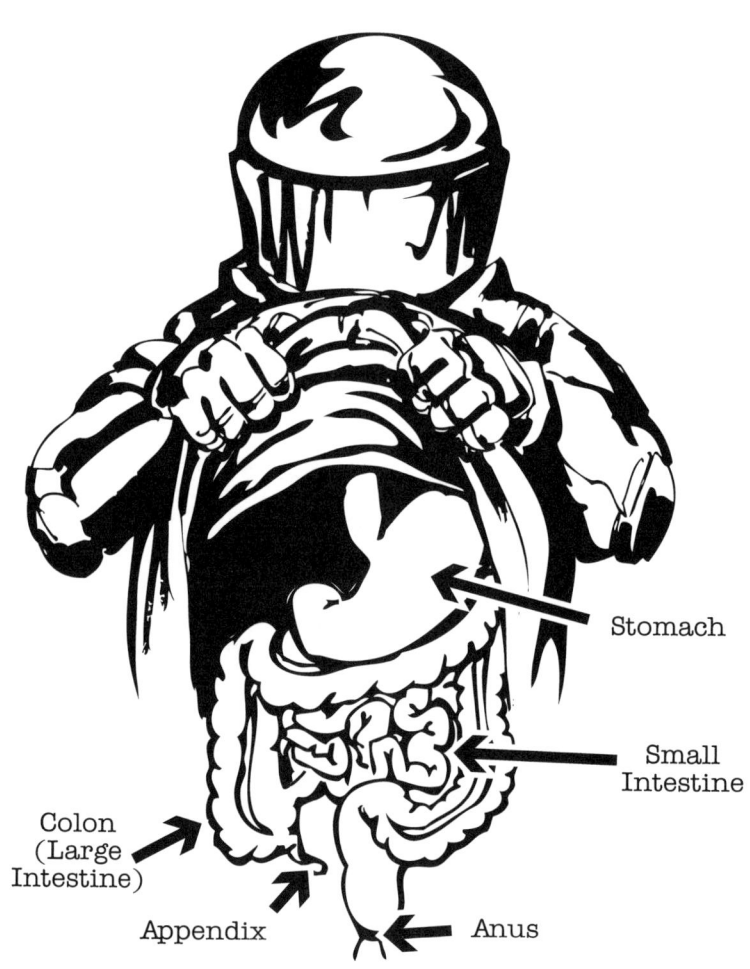

Stomach

Small
Intestine

Colon
(Large
Intestine)

Appendix

Anus

Your Gut Feelings Count

Sooner or later, one out of seven motorcyclists will get appendicitis. It's most common in men between the ages of 10 and 30, and is the most common cause for surgery on the abdomen. Since it's not unusual for doctors to miss it on the first visit to the office, being clued in to the symptoms makes it more likely that you'll get appropriate care sooner. And time, when it comes to appendicitis, is important.

The appendix is a small sac about the size of your pinkie finger, attached near the beginning of the large bowel (or colon) in the lower right part of your abdominal cavity. It's only open at the top and closed at the far end, and is called a "blind" sac. Its main purpose is providing boat payments for surgeons and anesthesiologists.

It becomes blocked on occasions, sometimes due to a "soft" obstruction (such as swelling of the lymph nodes or a piece of fecal material (medicalese for "poop"). By the time the pathologist opens the appendix, though, the "soft obstruction" is usually not seen. "Hard obstructions" can include seeds, fecaliths (tiny pieces of petrified poop—oops, I mean "fecal material") or even intestinal parasites like pinworms or roundworms. "Hard" obstructions get worse a lot quicker than "soft" obstructions do.

After it gets blocked, the appendix becomes inflamed. That's because the colon is full of fecal material, which is about 80 percent bacteria. When closed up in a small space, bacterial growth stretches the wall of the appendix, causing pain.

Though the appendix is in the right lower part of your abdomen, the initial pain often is in the midline. That's because the nerves to your appendix were formed while you were an embryo. Then, the appendix was part of a midline gut structure. These "visceral" (or gut) nerves respond mainly to stretching, and don't feel pain directly as the "somatic" or bodily nerves do.

Later, the inflammation spreads to the walls of the appendix, and irritates the walls of your abdominal cavity. Now, the abdominal walls have somatic nerves, which respond to all kinds of pain, and are pretty precise in "where" they feel stuff. Somatic nerves are the ones that go to the rest of your body (soma) rather than your innards (viscera). That's why the pain moves down to the right lower quadrant, to a spot called McBurney's point.

It's easy to find this point. Draw a line from the front part of the pelvic crest (you've got one on each side at about the height of your navel) to the middle of your pubic bone in the front. McBurney's Point is near the middle of this line, sometimes a little below it. Even early in appendicitis, deep pressure here will produce pain. Later on, even slight pressure or jiggling this area will hurt.

Since things that make the inflamed abdominal cavity scrape over the inflamed wall of the appendix cause pain, activities like coughing (which moves things in the abdomen) or bouncing up and down on your toes will hurt, too. These are pretty important signs, and if you find you're having typical symptoms (as listed below) that include this kind of pain, call your doctor or go to an emergency room. Don't wait, and don't eat or drink anything while waiting!

Unfortunately, appendicitis isn't always clear-cut. In infants, old people, women, immunosupressed patients, and folks who are on steroids, the picture can be confusing. However, here's a typical course of events:

First, you'll lose your appetite. You might eat, but you probably wouldn't eat much. Then, or a little later, you'd feel a vague pain in your mid-abdomen, typically in the neighborhood of your navel. Note; it's unusual for the pain to start in the right lower quadrant, but it might happen. *Remember: loss of appetite and abdominal pain should make you think "appendicitis."*

Usually, the pain later shifts to the right lower part of the abdomen. A low fever isn't uncommon; diarrhea or constipation also occur frequently. If it goes untreated, the appendix may rupture, spreading fecal bacteria (and infection) inside the abdominal cavity. This is called "peritonitis," since the infection is in the peritoneal cavity, lined by a thin layer called peritoneum. This is a Big Problem, and is best avoided. In cowboy movies, folks who were gut-shot died of peritonitis.

Not all inflamed appendices rupture if they go untreated. Occasionally, folks will have a mild episode of appendicitis that clears up on its own, and then comes back again weeks to months later. This might be due to the nature of the obstruction, which could be "soft," and come and go.

If the appendix ruptures, there may then be a brief period where the pain improves (due to lack of stretching of the appendix) but this is soon followed by peritonitis. If peritonitis goes untreated, it's likely to be fatal.

When diagnosed before it ruptures, the treatment of appendicitis is straightforward. You find a surgeon, and have him or her remove it. Nowadays, though, many appendices are being removed by laparascopic surgery, and a report ("Annals of Surgery," January, 2004) indicates this method may have advantages even in ruptured or perforated appendicitis. Patients went home sooner and were also less likely to need intensive care.

Making the diagnosis is much easier if you're male. You don't have a significant amount of other equipment in the area that can give similar symptoms. In women, an infection of the fallopian tube (pelvic inflammatory disease, or P.I.D.) is sometimes confused with appendicitis. It's now getting easier to diagnose appendicitis in unclear cases using ultrasound and CT (computerized tomography). Especially when using the compressibility test, sensitivity and specificity of ultrasound is high.

However, even using imaging procedures, appendicitis can be tough to diagnose. An employee at my office recently had abdominal pain that I thought was appendicitis. She went to the ER for blood tests, etc., and since the ultrasound and CT were both negative, she was sent home. Her pain persisted, so the surgeon operated, and guess what?

Appendicitis.

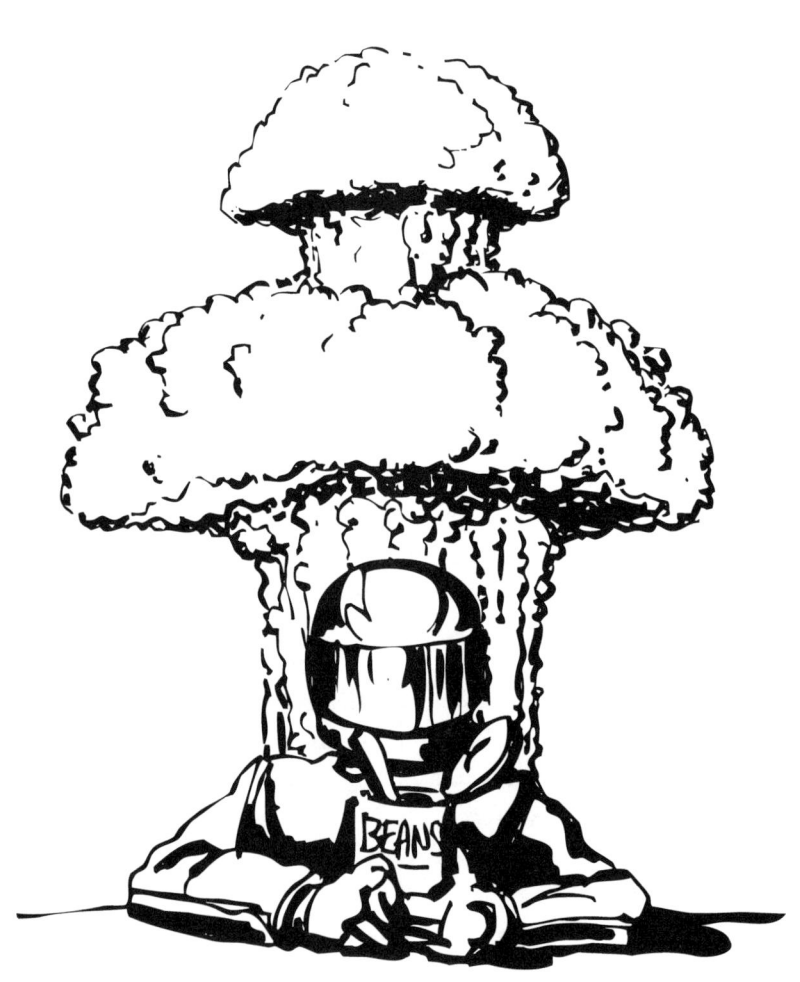

Farts

In cold weather, wearing a completely zipped-up Aerostich and then eating a lot of beans is a hazardous combination. A well-made riding suit negates one of the true joys of motorcycling—being able to fart with impunity. Windproof clothing can preserve farts longer than you'd expect. Arriving at someone's home, removing the 'Stich, and releasing the fumes can be embarrassing. Here's a suggestion—open the zipper for the last mile or so.

To tell the truth, human beings aren't responsible for farts. The bacteria that live in our colons are the culprits—they produce methane (AKA, swamp gas), hydrogen and mercaptans, among other gases, after metabolizing nutrients you didn't absorb. In other words, bacteria fart, not people.

Sadly, healthy diets can increase fart production. We all remember "Beans, beans, the musical fruit . . ." Beans cause farts because they contain certain oligosaccharides, which are sugar molecules that we can't break down, digest, and absorb. In addition to beans, other fruits and vegetables that contain oligosaccharides include cabbage, oats, wheat, chickpeas, peanuts, lentils, peas, soy-content foods, broccoli, Brussels sprouts, carrots, corn, leeks, onions, parsnips, and squash. For you Scrabble® fans, these oligosaccharides are raffinose, stachyose, and verbascose. Such complex sugars are combinations of simple sugars that we normally have no problem digesting, like fructose, sucrose, galactose and glucose. But since we can't absorb them, these complex sugars pass through the small intestine and end up in the colon, where the bacteria live.

Your colon makes up about the last 4 to 6 feet of your gut, and is packed with *E. coli* bacteria. More than three-quarters of the weight of each bowel movement is live bacteria—no, *umm*, kidding. These bacteria love raffinose, stachyose, and verbascose, and consequently, the bacteria fart up a storm when these nutrients arrive in the colon. Maybe the reason that these bacteria get away with farting so much is that it's dark inside your gut, and the other bacteria can't tell which bacterium is responsible, "Hey! Who did that?"

Some of a fart's nastiest smell components are mercaptans, which contain sulfur. Mercaptans also give natural gas its smell, and skunks use it in their, *umm,* perfume. When you eat foods with more sulfur, like eggs, cauliflower, and meat, more mercaptans are produced in your gut, causing the fart to smell much worse. Vegetarians (and vegetarian animals) tend to produce farts that aren't anywhere as pungent as carnivores' farts. Remember that when choosing a tent-mate.

Methane is common to all farts. Also, some substances in our food can pass unabsorbed completely through the digestive tract. Garlic, for example, contains substances that not only pass through your gut, but can even be found in your sweat if you eat enough of it. And though it has no odor, the nitrogen in the air many people swallow passes unchanged through the gut. And what goes in, must come out, as Fudd said.

If desired, you can prevent farts. I say, "if desired," because most guys will probably admit, if questioned using a lie detector, that they don't mind their own farts much. If you live alone in the wilderness and never see other human beings, controlling farts doesn't make much sense. For those of us who don't fit that description, here's one useful tip: Soak your beans overnight and change the water at least once. This will remove many of the beans' oligosaccharides, which will starve some of your gut bacteria.

Beano® is a good fart preventer. It contains an enzyme that breaks apart the oligosaccharides that your body otherwise couldn't digest; then, your own body can absorb the simple sugars that make them up. To use it, just add five drops to fart-producing food when you start your meal. It's important not to add it to food that's too hot to eat. You'll stop the action of the alpha-d-galactosidase enzyme, and it won't work. But when used properly, it's quite effective.

We men know that farting is one of mankind's oldest pleasures, and one of womankind's oldest gripes. I almost believe there's a Y-chromosome linked trait that lets men enjoy (or at least tolerate) farts—the absence of this gene leads to typical female repulsion. If you remember that wonderful scene from "Blazing Saddles," everyone around the campfire was male. (Note: This scene was sadly chopped from the television version.)

Here's more proof that there's a fundamental difference between the way men and women perceive farts. Many years ago, I felt a fart coming on. I said to my (then) girlfriend, "Listen!" I then proceeded to play the first seven notes of "Over the Rainbow," using mostly methane. I was delighted and proud—I hadn't played a wind instrument in years. She got up, got dressed, and left, and that was the end of the relationship. Go figure. Obviously, she didn't appreciate music.

On the other hand, farts can be good news, as anyone who's had intestinal surgery knows. After surgery, you won't get any food 'til you fart, which indicates that your gut is starting to work again.

The sociology of farts is interesting. We all know that after passing a silent fart we should look at someone else in the room, raise our eyebrows, and look away with a slightly pained expression. (Don't try this with only two people in the room.)

Another time-honored ploy is to say "Rex! Bad dog! Go outside!" shaking your head ruefully. This is a useful ploy, but you must know certain facts to make it work. First, the fart must have been silent (dog farts make no noise). Next, it requires the presence of a dog. If you try this on your cat, it will lose whatever little respect (if any) it has for you.

By the way, if "Rex" farts a lot, there's a version of Beano® that dogs can use. They like the taste, and it works very well. And it has the most perfect name of any consumer product I've ever encountered.

The product's called CurTail.

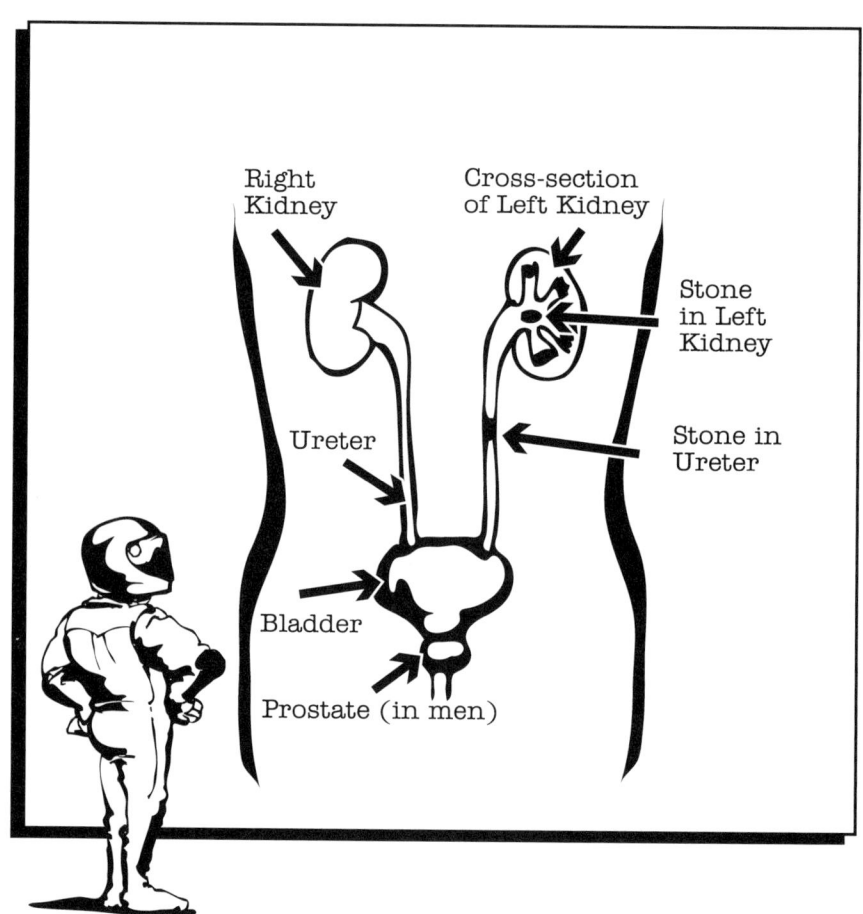

Right Kidney

Cross-section of Left Kidney

Stone in Left Kidney

Ureter

Stone in Ureter

Bladder

Prostate (in men)

Stoned

Kidney stones are one of the most painful conditions known to man. I say "man" because men are 2 to 3 times as likely to get kidney stones than are women. About one in eight male motorcyclists will get a stone, more than the number who'll get hit by an SUV. Most stones in the U.S. occur in white or Asian men between 20 and 49—it's less likely for them to start after 50.

Anatomy: You have two kidneys at the back of your abdominal cavity where your lower ribs join your spine. Each kidney filters waste products out of your blood and washes them away with water. Drinking more water is *easier* on your kidneys. When urine is dark and concentrated, crystals can form, eventually growing into kidney stones.

Calcium (75 percent), uric acid (6 percent), and cystine (2 percent) are the most common material in stones. Struvite stones (15 percent) are found mainly in women as a result of urinary tract infections. Some medications, like Indinavir (Crixivan) for HIV, can cause stones, too. Stones start microscopically small, and grow in the renal pelvis, which is the collecting area inside each kidney. When they break loose and head downstream, they go into the ureter, which connects the kidneys to the bladder. That's when the trouble starts.

The ureter is a narrow tube that's normally flat and closed, like an un-inflated balloon. When a stone is in the ureter, it often causes severe, crampy pain. The location depends on where the stone is. When close to the kidney, the pain is usually in the back. As it moves down the ureter, the pain is felt in the side or abdomen. Eventually, as it nears the bladder, pain is felt in the groin. When it's near the bladder, urinary symptoms (like urinating a lot) result.

The pain of a stone is often described like "a knife" or "the worst pain of my life." Patients with kidney stones often can't find a comfortable position. They'll walk around or move a lot if they're lying down. Another common symptom is nausea and vomiting. Most stones will cause some bleeding, though at times the bleeding can't be seen. However, about one in six stones cause no bleeding, even on microscopic analysis or laboratory testing.

If you've never had a kidney stone, the above symptoms need to be checked out by your doctor or an E.R. Emergency rooms see about a half-million kidney stone patients in the U.S. a year. The E.R. will make sure that the pain is indeed caused by a stone (instead of a dissecting abdominal aortic aneurysm, shingles, appendicitis, gall bladder disease, pancreatitis, pneumonia, bowel obstruction, testicular torsion, etc.); that you don't also have a urinary infection; and that the stone's not blocking the ureter, which can damage the kidney.

The best test is what's called a "spiral (or helical) CT" which can show most all stones, even the non-calcium ones that don't show up on plain X-rays. One of the few stones that doesn't show up on CT is caused by Indinavir (Crixivan). If you're taking it and have unexplained abdominal pain, make sure to tell the clinician you see (and remind her of this fact). Often, the doctor will order a plain abdominal X-ray (i.e., a "flat plate" of the abdomen) since once a stone is identified, following its progress using plain films is a lot easier (and cheaper).

If you just have a stone, it's likely that you'll get some morphine or Toradol for pain, and be given an IV to help increase your urine flow, which might wash the stone down into the bladder. When you're sent home, you'll probably be given some narcotic pain medicine for severe pain, such as Vicodin or Percocet, as well as an anti-inflammatory like Aleve (naproxen) or ibuprofen. Two other drugs that may be helpful are nifedipine, a blood pressure medication that relaxes smooth muscle (like that in blood and the wall of the ureter) and prednisone, which can shrink inflamed tissue in the ureter, helping the stone pass.

If the stone needs to be removed, there are several ways to do it. Extracorporeal shock wave lithotripsy (ESWL) uses an underwater energy wave that's focused on the stone, and can shatter it into fragments small enough to pass through the ureter. It works best on stones smaller than about 2.5cm, and is most useful when used on stones above the level of the pelvis. About two thirds of stones can be treated with ESWL.

Another way stones are removed is by using a flexible instrument called a ureterscope that's passed up into the bladder and then into the ureter. If the stone is small enough (under about 5mm) it can be grabbed and pulled out. If it's larger, it can be pushed higher so ESWL can be used, or sometimes broken up and removed through the ureterscope.

For larger stones; those that fail ESWL; those that are either in the kidney or high in the ureter; and those causing obstruction, a urologist can make a puncture through the flank and into the kidney. Using this technique, the stone can be removed, and the kidney can be allowed to drain. It's also useful for people in whom ESWL is contraindicated, such as pregnant women. If the obstruction isn't relieved, permanent kidney damage will result.

After being diagnosed with a kidney stone, it's very helpful to find out what kind of stone it is. Typically, you'll be given a special strainer to urinate through. If you catch the stone, it can be analyzed and treatment can be individualized to prevent them in the future. But no matter what kind of stone it is, drinking more water helps. The ideal urine output is 2 to 3 liters a day—that is about 4 to 6 pints, or half to three quarters of a gallon. Since the bladder holds about a pint, that means urinating about 4 to 6 times a day. And if you've ever suffered through a kidney stone, drinking the extra water—more if it's hot and/or dry—is well worth it.

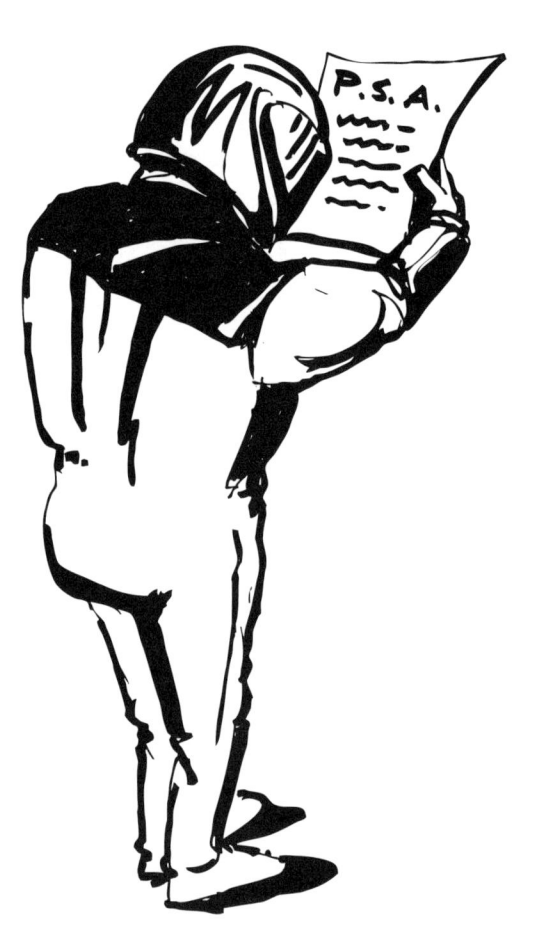

For Men Only

There's more to being a man than liking gadgets, owning fast machinery, and being unable to ask directions—some body parts define us as males. Since these parts spend lives closer to our motorcycles than any other organs, they're very appropriate topics for this book.

Male-specific parts include the penis, testicles, and prostate. We're all familiar with the penis and testes. The prostate, though, is a vague "something down there" when we're young, and a subject of growing concern as we age.

The prostate makes some of the fluid in semen, helping transport sperm. It's a shy and retiring organ, at least compared to the penis. Located in front of the rectum and below the bladder, a normal prostate's about the size and shape of a walnut. It wraps around the urethra, the tube connecting the bladder to the outside world, so prostate problems often affect the flow of urine.

There are three common prostate problems—prostatitis (infection/inflammation/pain); benign prostatic hypertrophy (overgrowth); and prostate cancer.

When your prostate's painful, infected, and/or inflamed, it's called prostatitis. About half of all men get it at least once, either acutely (suddenly) or chronically (lingering). Testing for prostatitis includes checking urine that's obtained before and after the physician massages the prostate. Sometimes, the secretions that are pushed out of the prostate are checked. These specimens are examined microscopically and cultured to see if bacteria or white blood cells are present. There's concern that pressure on an acutely inflamed and infected prostate could push microbes into the bloodstream—in acute prostatitis, a physician might choose to not massage the prostate to collect secretions.

Acute prostatitis often has a sudden onset, with fever, chills, pain on urination, urinary urgency, or inability to urinate (which is guaranteed to make somebody get medical care, fast). Since symptoms of prostatitis can resemble those of a urinary tract infection (UTI), information that helps tell them apart is useful. Here's a clue that may be helpful—in prostatitis, the color of the semen when you ejaculate may be darker than usual. Sometimes it's yellow or green. In a urinary infection, there won't be any change in semen color. Also, in prostatitis, ejaculation may hurt, which it shouldn't with just a UTI. If you notice this happening (discolored semen or painful ejaculation) be sure to tell your doctor, even without other symptoms.

Acute prostatitis is treated with antibiotics, but often needs a long course of treatment—I always treat it for at least a month, since better initial treatment might keep acute prostatitis from becoming chronic prostatitis. If acute prostatitis gets better with antibiotics, I try to treat for at least 2 to 4 weeks longer, which may help eradicate it.

Chronic prostate pain problems are very common—unfortunately, it's not clear just what causes them. Though some seem to be due to bacterial infection, and there are cases that respond to antibiotics, in many other cases repeated doses of antibiotics don't do much, if any, good.

Symptoms are often vague or even absent in chronic prostatitis. Men will sometime have pain behind their scrotum, back pain, sudden need to urinate, an unexplained fever, or low abdominal pain. It, too, can also cause pain on ejaculation.

Research shows that some chronically painful prostates show inflammation, while others don't. Treatment is controversial. There may be a connection between prostatitis and prostate cancer. This is still being looked at. Some evidence suggests that evidence of inflammation is linked to cancer later.

Prostate cancer can often be detected by physical exam (which is one reason why older men need regular physicals), ultrasound, and through the P.S.A. test. (P.S.A. stands for prostate-specific antigen, and is higher in prostate cancer and in men with a large or inflamed prostate.)

Prostate cancer usually occurs in older men, though Frank Zappa died of it at 52. As men age, the likelihood of getting diagnosed with PrCa increases—about 2/3rds of men who reach 80 will have evidence of it in their prostate gland. Since it usually grows very slowly, more men die *with* it than *from* it. Because of this slow growth rate, there has been controversy on whether using screening blood tests like PSA is worthwhile.

In a man whose expected lifespan is relatively short (say, definitely less than ten years), who has no prostate symptoms like impaired urine flow, some physicians argue against doing a PSA test. The reasoning is that a slow-growing tumor that's too small to cause symptoms now probably won't kill the person before they die. On the other hand, if a man's got a family history of PrCa or breast cancer, and has more than ten years to live, screening makes more sense.

Just because prostate cancer is usually slow growing doesn't mean it can't cause problems. I had a patient whose prostate cancer had spread to his spine and rib cage. Not only did he have continuous bone pain, but the tumor had invaded his bone marrow, causing anemia. It also caused paralysis of one of his legs. Regular screening probably would have prevented this.

If detected early, prostate cancer can be treated with good success and often can be completely cured. Treatment is either surgical, radiation, and/or chemotherapy. There's a lot of controversy whether surgery is preferable to radiation, since there are pluses and minuses to each approach. That's why some men, like Bob Dole, Colin Powell, John Kerry, and Norman Schwarzkopf chose surgery, and Rupert Murdoch, Charlton Heston, Rudolph Giuliani, and Nelson Mandela went with radiation. Some men didn't get the cancer detected in time, like Frank Zappa, Telly Savalas, and Timothy Leary—they died of the disease.

The take-home message is to get your prostate checked at least annually once you reach 50 (or 40 if you're African-American or have a strong family history of prostate or breast cancer). Remember, after you hit 40, your warranty expires. And after you're fifty, you can't even find replacement parts . . .

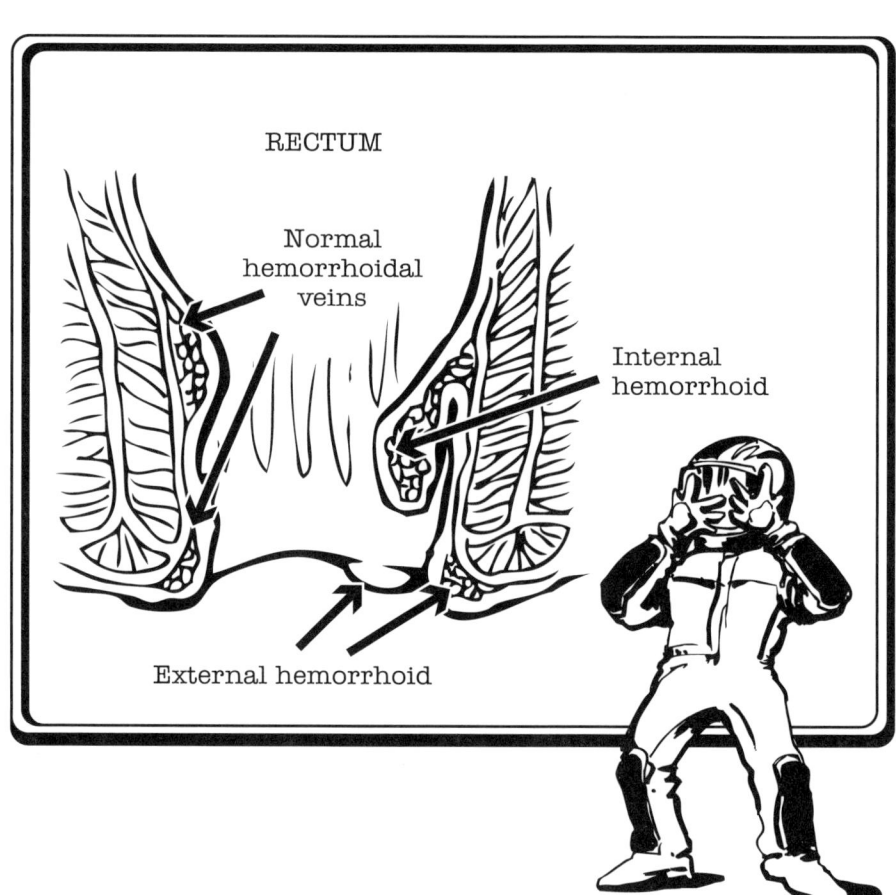

Hemorrhoids

It's said that to be a successful political leader, one needs "glasses for the look of intelligence, white hair for the look of sincerity, and hemorrhoids for the look of concern."

Hemorrhoids are no laughing matter. Napoleon may have lost the Battle of Waterloo because his hemorrhoids kept him up the night before. If you've experienced hemorrhoids, I'm sure you can sympathize.

Motorcyclists are at high risk for hemorrhoids. We spend hours sitting; some of us don't exercise much; and we often have poor diets when on the road.

If you haven't had hemorrhoids yet, there's a good chance you will. And take my word for it—having them will change your motorcycling experience in a "fundamental" way. If you'd like to avoid them, this article will teach you how. If you've got them, you'll learn to deal with them.

What are hemorrhoids? Functionally, they're just veins, like varicose veins. When you bear down, increasing the pressure in your abdomen, pressure in your hemorrhoidal veins increase too, making them bulge. They come in three flavors (oops—bad choice of words); internal, external, and mixed.

Mixed hemorrhoids are a combination of an internal and external hemorrhoid.

External hemorrhoids feel like bulges outside the anus that bulge out more after a bowel movement. At that time, applying pressure to empty them of blood is a good idea. The surface of an external hemorrhoid has nerves. If you touch it, you'll feel it.

Internal hemorrhoids start completely above the rectum. They don't have nerves.

Sometimes, internal hemorrhoids can "prolapse" or hang out through the rectum. When they do this, they're more likely to bleed. Their surface is delicate, and often gets irritated when it's rubbed with plain, dry toilet paper. If your hemorrhoids are irritated, use wet TP or wet wipes, followed with gentle blotting.

Another good option is using the shower (Note: Avoid soap, washcloths, or *anything* except plain water) after a BM.

Hemorrhoids often get worse during pregnancy, when the swollen womb pushes on the blood vessels returning to the heart; during coughing, when each cough increases pressure throughout the venous system; when spending too much time on the toilet; with some liver problems; and when bowel movements are too hard, requiring extra pressure.

Very often, hemorrhoids are first found when they start to bleed. Hemorrhoidal bleeding is usually bright red, sometimes dripping or even squirting into the toilet. However, if the blood is dark or mixed with stool, the problem may be higher in the colon. Get it checked! It may be a sign of colon or rectal cancer.

Softening the stool is critical in preventing and treating hemorrhoids. Soft stool needs less pushing; consequently, there's less bulging and less possibility of . . .

Thrombosed Hemorrhoids

Since hemorrhoids are full of blood, sometimes they clot, exemplifying the term "pain in the butt." If small, they hurt for several days, during which time you can count on "the look of concern" being present almost continuously. This sensation gradually fades, typically lasting about a week, as your body absorbs the clot.

While your hemorrhoids are acting up, avoid heavy lifting. When lifting, many people "grunt" and increase the pressure in the abdomen (which also stabilized the trunk). When abdominal pressure increases, the pressure on the veins increases too. This may make hemorrhoids worse.

Treatment for thrombosed hemorrhoids is a combination of stool softeners like Colace® (docusate) or fiber like Metamucil® (psyllium) and *plenty* of extra fluids—an extra 6 to 8 glasses a day is a good idea. The extra fluid will soften the bowel movement. Take it from me—you'll never appreciate a soft BM as much as when you have a thrombosed hemorrhoid.

A newer treatment is using Diosmin, which is a plant-derived bioflavonoid that is very helpful both for hemorrhoids and for treatment after hemorrhoid surgery. Diosmin is available online, though the form used in most studies is produced by Servier, a French company, and may not be available in the U.S. This substance increases venous tone (i.e., helps tighten veins) and has been shown to help both hemorrhoids as well as other problems, like venous leg ulcers.

A mild pain medication is often needed (an over-the-counter med such as Tylenol®, Advil®, or Aleve® provides pain relief without constipation), and importantly, sitz baths. How do you do sitz baths? Simple! Just put a few inches of hot water into the bathtub, and you sitz in the bath several times daily. This both cleans and soothes the anal area.

Don't use laxatives when you have a thrombosed hemorrhoid. Even though constipation is bad, diarrhea can be worse. Remember, stool softeners are *not* laxatives.

Surgery

In the first three days, the surgical treatment for thrombosed hemorrhoids is numbing up the skin with xylocaine, cutting off the top, and then lifting out the clot that's causing the problem. If older than three days, stool softening measures and sitz baths several times a day are used. Severe internal hemorrhoids are sometimes treated by injection (which clots them so they fall off; banding (a tight rubber band around the base "chokes" them, and they fall off); and sometimes other treatments, like cutting them out or burning them off. Unfortunately, treatment is often quite painful, and may cause other problems, too.

Prevention

The best way to prevent (and to treat) hemorrhoids is by having only soft BMs. Colace® (docusate) is a good softener, and you can get fiber from vegetables and fruit; from commercial bulk laxatives like Metamucil®; and from bran, which is in many breakfast cereals. You can tell if you're getting enough roughage by the, *umm,* end result. Exercise, a good diet, healthy bowel habits, and getting those magazines out of the bathroom should go a long way in preventing them.

The Bottom Line

Hemorrhoids are a common problem among motorcyclists, as well as the general public. Keep in mind that it's *especially* important to prevent hemorrhoids, since you only have one *. (Note: read the last sentence out loud).

Concerns
on Long Trips

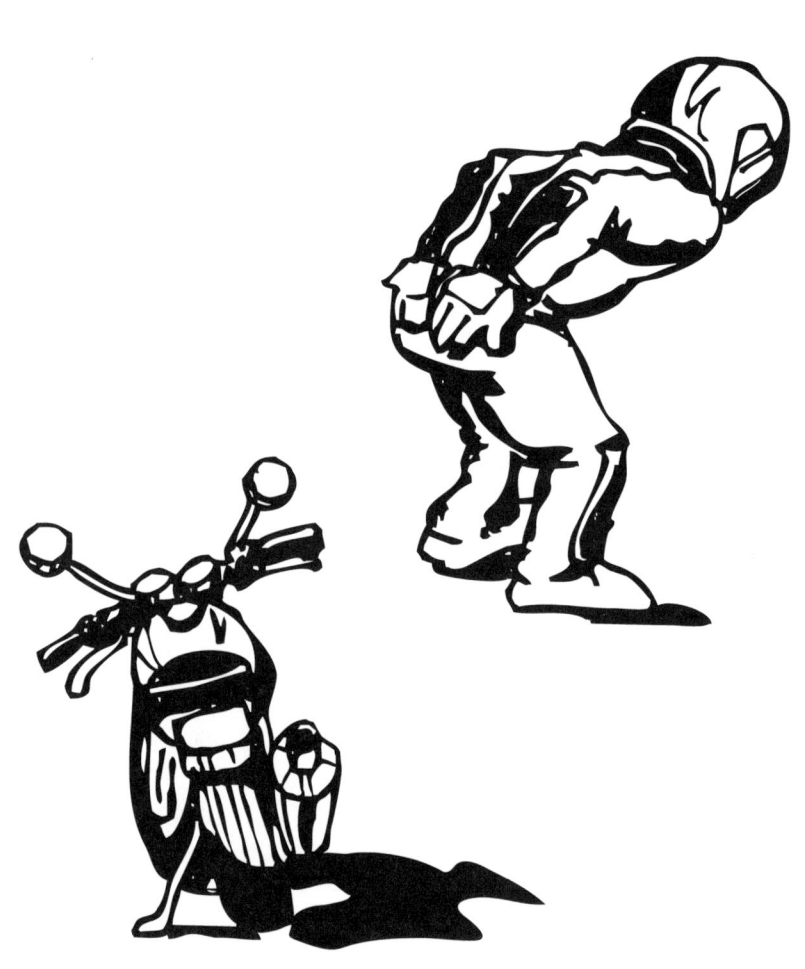

Monkey Butt

If your butt or inner thighs have ever been sore and red after a long, hot ride, you've suffered from monkey butt. It happens when the skin breaks down from friction, pressure, and moisture. Since we all sit on our butts most of the time that we're riding (and you trials riders can just sit down and be qu—oops—no, you can't really sit down, can you?), factors affecting our butts are of fundamental (so to speak) importance.

The top layer of your skin is called the stratum corneum or horny layer. "Cornu" is Latin for horn, and horn contains keratin, a tough substance that's also in fingernails, toenails, hair, feathers, hooves and the outer layer of skin. Hence, horny layer. It's there for protection and abrasion resistance.

When your skin gets moist, this layer gets soft. Think of what happens to the hard skin on your heels after a hot shower or a long bath. You can rub it right off with your fingers. When the protective layer gets soft, it loses its protective qualities and the skin becomes more vulnerable. In order to preserve this protective layer, the skin must be kept dry.

The best way to do this is to either leave the skin totally exposed to air or to have a wicking layer of fabric next to your skin. Since riding naked isn't a viable option for most of us, wearing fabric that doesn't get damp is the best plan. For years, I've only worn synthetic fiber underwear from www.Wickers.com—they make specially designed fabrics designed to pull the moisture away from your skin and let it evaporate (and they've got outstanding customer service and excellent products). They've even got underwear with no seams on the area you sit on, which is ideal for motorcyclists.

Synthetic fibers are much better than cotton when it comes to moisture transport. Cotton absorbs moisture initially, but the moisture stays in the fabric. The material gets damp and keeps the moisture next to the skin. When it does, the keratin layer of your skin gets soft and loses its protective qualities, letting the pressure and friction damage the skin.

Since synthetic fabrics resist getting moist, they keep you cool and dry when it's hot, and warm and dry when it's cold. In any condition, wet fabric next to your skin is a Bad Thing. Possibly as a result of only using synthetics against my skin—never cotton—I've never had a trace of monkey butt, even after 12-hour days in hot weather. My shirts are synthetic fiber, too—I won't wear anything else.

Another effective strategy to minimize friction and moisture is to use a specialized powder. In 2003, Andy Thompson and Dr. Greg Burroughs, both motorcyclists, came up with Anti Monkey Butt powder (www.antimonkeybutt.com). It's a mixture of talc, the best drying agent for the skin, and calamine, which soothes and helps healing.

Don't use baby powder for this. It's made of cornstarch, which is good at absorbing moisture, but can contribute to the yeast growth—Not A Good Thing down there. Cornstarch is in baby powder since it's safer for babies to breathe than talc, but for men—talc is better. Note: Talc is statistically linked with ovarian cancer. The women at higher risk for cancer had used talc more than 10,000 times, directly on the perineum or on a diaphragm.

Calamine, the other ingredient in Anti Monkey Butt powder, is zinc oxide with a little ferric oxide for color. Zinc oxide is white, ferric oxide (rust) is red—together, they're pink. Calamine has been used for decades (remember *Poison Ivy* by the Coasters from 1959? "You're gonna need an ocean of calamine lotion . . .") and is great for your skin. The combination should be very effective. I'm told that AMB powder is also popular with long distance truckers and with electricians, since both have sweaty jobs.

A third factor to prevent monkey butt is a seat that fits correctly. If a seat fits right, you can ride all day without any discomfort. When there's a mismatch between your seat and your butt, some areas will carry more of the weight than others. Typically, the ischial tuberosities (those are the bones in your butt that you feel if you sit on your hands) take most of the pressure. If the pressure on the skin is more than the pressure in the blood vessels, blood won't flow and that skin doesn't get any oxygen, effectively strangling it. This results in pain, irritation, and skin damage. When this happens to an area of skin, it's called a "hot spot."

A good saddle distributes your weight so you don't get hot spots. The late, great Bill Mayer was a pioneer in custom saddles—three of the best custom saddlemakers on the planet use his techniques. His sons, Rick Mayer (530-357-BUTT / 530-357-2888) and Rocky Mayer (800-242-ROCKY / 800-242-7625), have carried on the family tradition, and I've heard many good things about their work. Russell Day-Long Saddles (800-4-DAY-LONG / 800-432-9566) uses technology invented and sold to them by Bill Mayer before Bill started his own company again.

I don't think you can go wrong with a custom saddle by any of these folks. They all guarantee your satisfaction. When Bill Mayer made my current saddle (one of the best investments I've ever made in a motorcycle accessory) I rode up to his shop so he could custom carve it. He carved a saddle blank so it was a good fit, covered it with plastic, and said "go ride for an hour or so." When I returned, I pointed out areas where I felt more pressure than other places and he shaved them down. I repeated this process a couple of times until it was perfect.

Now I've got a saddle that fits my butt perfectly, and the fabric I'm sitting on stays dry for hours. Consequently, after an all-day ride, my butt never crosses my mind. And you just can't argue with the end result.

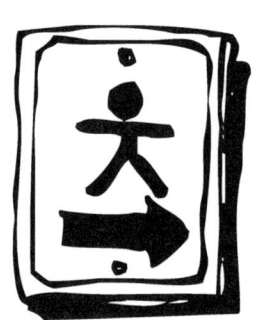
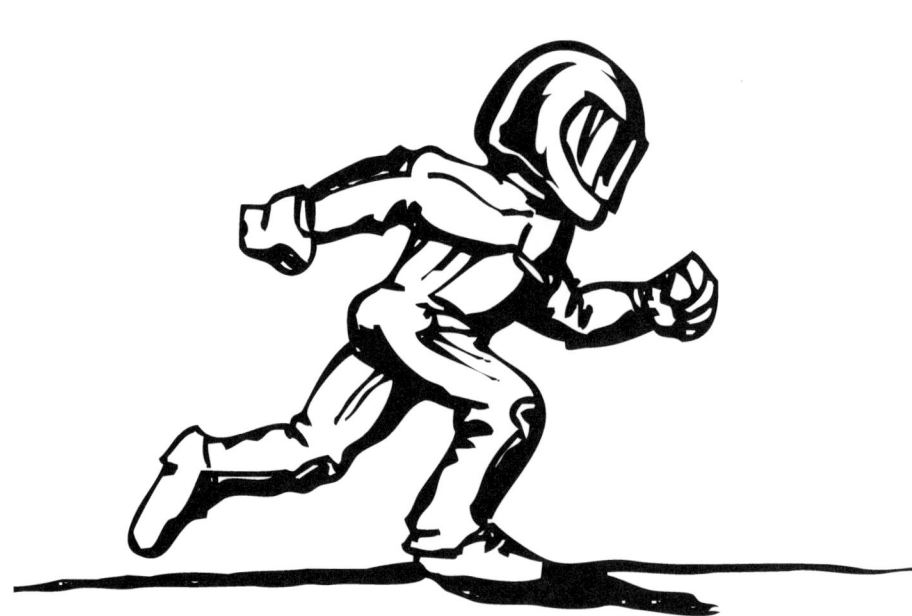

Born to Run

You don't want to see NEXT SERVICES 149 MILES when your gut starts gurgling. Nothing cramps riding plans—or your guts—like Montezuma's revenge, stomach flu, Delhi belly, food poisoning, the Aztec two-step, or "la turista."

These conditions are often preventable, and when they happen, there are good, and bad, treatments. Some people are a higher risk, too. First, let's talk prevention.

Most acute diarrheal illnesses are due to microorganisms, such as bacteria, viruses, or protozoans (like amoeba, as in "amoebic dysentery," or giardia). In some cases, they get into your food and grow, giving off byproducts (AKA "germ poop"), which make you sick. When this happens, the toxin (poison) is in the food, so the resultant illness is called "food poisoning." These toxins often survive cooking temperatures that will kill the bacteria themselves. One of the most common forms is staph food poisoning, which can be prevented by proper food handling.

Staph germs can be anywhere, especially in skin infections, like the skinned knuckle you got from adjusting the preload on your shock, or the little burn from your muffler, which you got adjusting the rebound. (Hint: Unless you're less of a klutz than I am, just keep your gloves on.) Staph germs like infecting food, so it's vital to keep sores, cuts, and burns from touching food that's being prepared unless it will be eaten within minutes. Staph toxin causes nasty, but usually short-lived, food poisoning, typically 4 to 6 hours after eating the bad food. It starts with cramps, followed by watery diarrhea, and is usually better in a day or so. You don't get fever with staph food poisoning.

Staph won't grow at less than 40° F or more than 140° F, so temperatures between these are called the "danger zone." Staph infect meat and dairy (think mayo in coleslaw or potato salad). If you doggie bag your lunch leftovers for dinner, you're at risk if they're not kept cold—don't just stick' em in the tankbag.

In food infections, as opposed to food poisoning, germs enter your body and grow, infecting you. They may be in the food; in the water used to clean or prepare it; or on the hand of the person cooking or serving it. That's why every restaurant bathroom reminds employees to wash their hands. If a few of an employee's normal gut germs (the *E. coli*) get on your drink can, they get on your hand when you touch it. When you then pick up your sandwich, you eat her *E. coli*. And *salmonella, shigella, campylobacter, amoeba, cholera,* and other nasties get passed on the same way.

Some areas have poor sanitation, poor food handling, and/or poor water supplies. They're typically in second- or third-world countries, but you're also at risk in some areas of the U.S. If you have doubts about the local sanitation, a good rule of thumb is to boil it, cook it, peel it, or forget it. Even so, cooking doesn't destroy staph toxin—if the meat was left out too long before cooking, it may be bad (but you can't taste it). Taking Pepto-Bismol with each meal lowers your risk—I use the tablets when traveling. And if going overseas, ask your doc about Rifaximin, a new antibiotic specific for travelers' diarrhea.

Once you've come down with the runs, what next? Don't start gobbling Imodium® or Lomotil®. Though either will likely stop the runs, that may not be what's best for you. Keep in mind that your body is producing diarrhea because of infection, inflammation, or irritation—you might be better off letting your body get rid of the bad stuff. And in some cases, you're a lot better off with antibiotics than with antidiarrheals. I suggest Imodium® or Lomotil® only for two things—when you can't stay near a bathroom for a day or so, or when you're having painful abdominal cramping. And when using these drugs, start with half a pill. Taking two at once, as often recommended, can turn your poop to plaster, so to speak. And that's a bad thing.

Now, if you've got a fever of 102° F, bloody diarrhea, or more than a couple of days of the runs, you need to see a doctor. If you can't keep any liquids down because of vomiting, ditto. Same if you take diuretics (water pills) or have a serious medical condition. Black or maroon stools are another danger sign—you may be bleeding internally.

But if you're less ill, with just cramps, diarrhea, and maybe a little vomiting, then what? The most important thing is to not get dehydrated, and/or low in certain blood chemicals called "electrolytes," like sodium or potassium. In some environments, like the Southwest U.S. in summer, you can get dehydrated without being sick. When you start to feel thirsty, you're already dry. Experienced riders drink enough fluids (other than caffeinated or alcoholic beverages, which dehydrate you) to urinate every four hours or less. Getting the runs in this environment can dehydrate you rapidly. Watch your urine color. If it's dark, you're low on water. A grumbling gut often occurs before diarrhea. Once you feel this, fluid is accumulating in your intestines. That's the time to start drinking more fluid, since the gut draws fluid from your bloodstream. You get dehydrated before the runs start.

Diarrhea contains electrolytes including sodium and potassium. If we lose 'lytes and only replace water, the concentration of these critical chemicals in our body decreases. This causes weakness, muscle cramps, and other problems. Fluids like fruit juice or electrolyte replacement drinks (Gatorade, etc.) will provide potassium and other necessary electrolytes. It's a good idea, though, to drink *both* water and electrolyte-containing drinks. And if small children get the runs, the electrolyte replacements sold in pharmacies (like PediaLyte) are even better. (The info here's aimed at adults, not kids.)

If you can't keep fluids down due to vomiting, just swallow one teaspoon per minute of juice or water. This almost always stays down, and helps prevent dehydration, which itself can cause nausea. When severe, dehydration can cause heart rhythm changes, weakness, and sometimes death. Prevention is key.

Remember: Don't Go Down From Condition Brown.

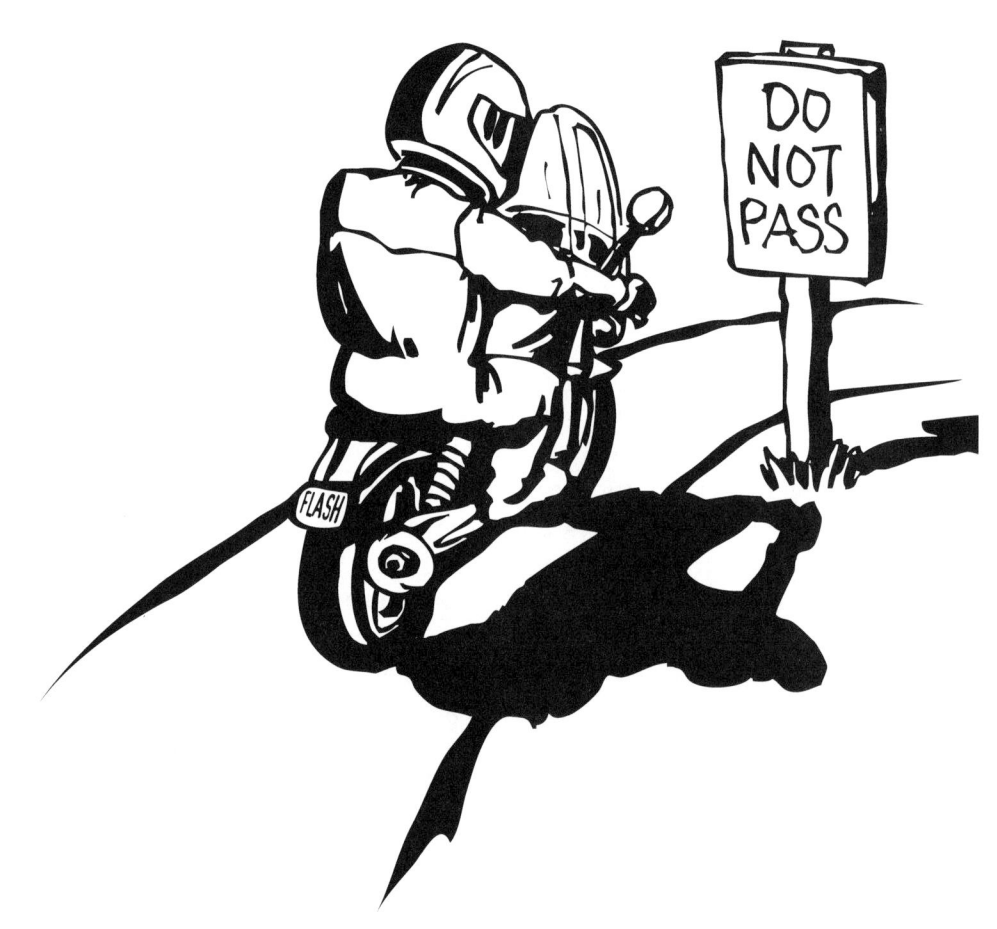

Constipation:
The Straight Poop

You've heard it said many times, "You are what you eat." This isn't quite true—you are what you eat, and *don't eliminate*. And if you're not eliminating, you're constipated. Four million Americans say they're constipated most or all of the time. Poor diet and/ or lack of exercise, two occurrences that often occur during some of my motorcycle trips, are common causes of constipation.

Other factors also contribute to the condition. If riders are rushing to get an early start, they might ignore their gut telling them to take a bathroom break. This is bad, because the longer stool stays in the gut, the drier and harder it becomes. The end result can be painful. If riders understand how their gut works, it's easy to prevent and treat its problems. Here's an overview on how your body processes food.

Your body is a hollow tube, topologically—similar to a doughnut. Food and drink enter the north end, and stool (and urine) exit from down south. What happens to the food in-between is digestion and excretion.

When you chew, you mix food with saliva, which has several enzymes. These start breaking down some of the food even before it reaches your stomach. Here's a demonstration of how these enzymes work. Chew a piece of bread for about a minute, and note how it starts tasting sweet. An enzyme in your saliva is breaking the starch in the bread down into sugar. The saliva also contains mucus, which lubricates the food and holds it together, making it easier to swallow.

When you swallow, food is propelled down your esophagus, which connects your mouth to your stomach. Once it gets to the stomach, food is churned and mixed with other digestive enzymes, and the stomach lining adds acid. The resultant liquid is called "chyme." Later, bile that's made in your liver and stored in the gall bladder, and digestive enzymes from the pancreas are added to this mix.

After leaving your stomach, the chyme enters your small intestine where the nutrients are absorbed. When the chyme finally arrives at the beginning of your large bowel, or colon, there are still several quarts of liquid remaining, along with the fiber and whatever else your body couldn't absorb. The walls of your colon are designed to absorb the liquid in the chyme, so you don't lose quarts of water each day. Not only would this be inconvenient, but it could also rapidly lead to dehydration. Dehydration due to diarrhea is one of the world's leading causes of death in children and infants. Your gut's goal is to produce stool with a proper consistency—dense enough to stick together, but soft enough that your gut can move it along and eventually eliminate it.

The contents of the gut move by peristalsis, or rhythmic contractions of the muscles in the gut wall. Some medications slow or stop this movement, which is needed to push the chyme and stool along. Medicines that slow the gut include narcotics, such as codeine, hydrocodone (found in Vicodin) and narcotic analogues such as Imodium and Lomotil. The latter two are made to treat diarrhea, but they may be stronger than desired. Because of this, individuals should take half the recommended dose. If it is absolutely necessary to use them, start taking psyllium (as in Metamucil) and drinking fluids immediately to prevent extreme constipation. Psyllium encourages regrowth of normal gut germs. Other medications causing constipation include iron supplements, some antacids, antidepressants, antispasmodics, diuretics, and anticonvulsants for epilepsy.

The slower the passage of the gut's contents, the more time your colon has to remove the water. If too much water is removed, the result is hard, dry stool, which can be painful—or in some cases impossible—to eliminate. A relative lack of physical activity can slow the transit of material through the gut, too. If you're normally fairly active but spend all day sitting on a motorcycle during a road trip, you might slow down your gut enough to produce constipation.

So, how is constipation treated? There are lots of preparations on the drugstore's shelves, but they fall into five major classes, all of which have different uses.

First are fiber laxatives, like psyllium (i.e., Metamucil® and in PerDiem Plain®). These prevent constipation by feeding normal gut germs, adding bulk. They're not good for individuals who are already constipated. I take PerDiem Plain on road trips where my diet's often poor and my exercise is minimal.

Next are stool softeners like Colace® and Surfak®. These add moisture, which can prevent stool from getting too hard. However, once you're already bound up, these may not help.

The third class are stimulant laxatives, such as Dulcolax®, Correctol®, Feen-A-Mint®, and Senokot®. These make the large bowel contract, which can get things moving again. Prunes fall into the same category as these drugs, and may help relieve constipation after it occurs. However, they shouldn't be used too often, since chronic use can lead to dependence.

Lubricants act like, well, lubricants. Mineral oil is the most common. It works by greasing the outside of the stool, allowing it to pass down (and hopefully out of) your gut. These can be helpful in relieving constipation too.

Saline laxatives (also called "osmotic" laxatives) are the most powerful. These act by bringing liquid through the walls of the gut into its inside, which moistens hard, dry stool and can help tremendously. Haley's M-O®, Milk of Magnesia, and Citrate of Magnesia® are all effective, though Citrate of Magnesia® is the most effective. If you use these, make sure you have access to the bathroom when they start working. Polyethylene glycol powder is a great product, since it's extremely powerful *and* gentle. However, it may take a few days to work. It's the best thing I've found for both preventing and relieving constipation, but it's prescription only.

Some of these medications are available in suppository form. Glycerin is a lubricant, which can help with very hard, dry stool. Dulcolax® contains biscodyl, which stimulates the colon and rectum (the last bit of colon before the anus). Other useful preparations are available as small, disposable enema kits. These include phospho-soda and mineral oil. Remember, if using an enema, lay on your left side. If this thought is unpleasant, just remember that an ounce of prevention is worth a pound of cure.

Effect of Emotions on Riding

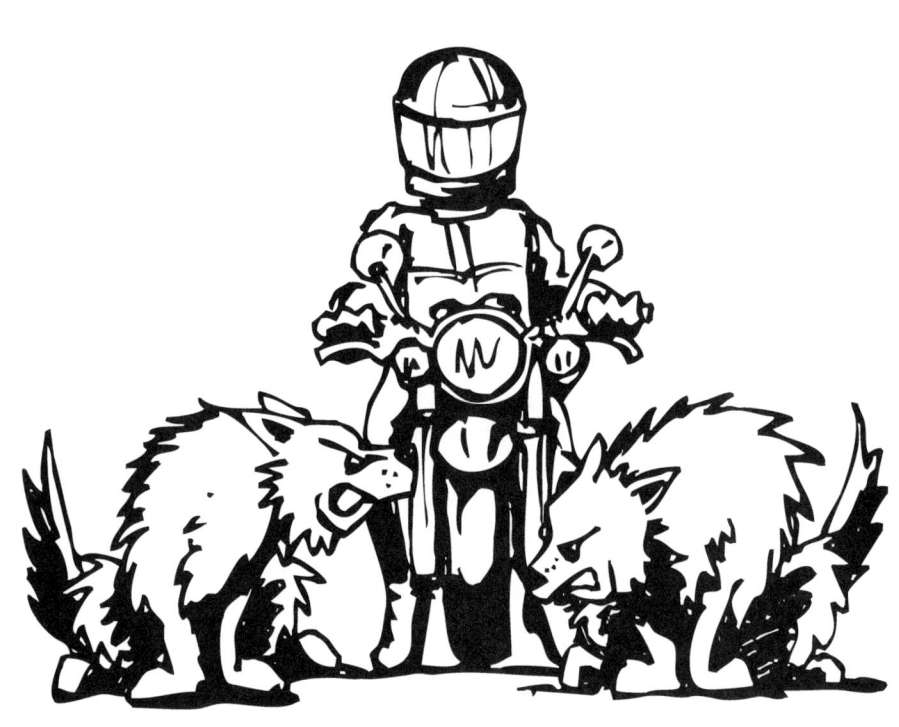

Testosterone Poisoning

Has this happened to you? You're riding along and an SUV blows past. You feel a surge of anger (Oh yeah?!) and immediately pass the SUV, perhaps giving him a 20 percent wave as you do so. You have a feeling of power and satisfaction as the SUV recedes rapidly in the mirror, only to be replaced by an "Oh, sh*t!" feeling when the highway patrol crests the hill ahead and hits his lights. You've just been a victim of testosterone poisoning (DWT—driving while 'testosteronified').

Testosterone is a male sex hormone (okay, a group of hormones, but I'll call them all "testosterone") that's associated with "male" behavior, including competitiveness, anger, and dominance. When we anticipate a competitive situation, testosterone levels rise. Testosterone reinforces behavior that is designed to "dominate" another individual. Testosterone also helps "bulk up" muscles—that's why some body-builders take steroid hormones (and sometimes, with excessive levels, they can become hyper-aggressive and get premature heart disease as well as liver problems).

However, there's evidence that aggressive behavior isn't a result of high testosterone. The behavior may actually be the cause of the higher hormone level, not the opposite. In one study, researchers put monkeys into a group and let them establish the "pecking order"—that is, monkey number one was "top dog" (top monkey?) and could grab the food and otherwise give a hard time to monkeys of lower rank; monkey number two could boss around all the other monkeys except number one, and so on.

The researchers gave extra testosterone to monkey number four, who normally only was "superior" to monkeys ranked 5 and below. He never gave monkeys one to three a hard time. After the testosterone, monkey four became a real bastard to monkeys 5 and below; but interestingly, he still kowtowed to one, two, and three. If testosterone caused aggressive behavior, you'd expect four to challenge one, two or three. He didn't. Testosterone seems to facilitate being aggressive, not cause it. So what causes aggression?

Let's think about the SUV. What we do depends on what we've learned earlier in life. In elementary school, I was the smallest (and usually the smartest) kid in my class. As a result, I got picked on. I stopped it by learning some judo and responding aggressively. Sometimes, I feel like I'm getting "picked on" while riding. "That SUV driver's dissing me!" and I respond by riding too aggressively. Take my word for it—this kind of behavior can have negative consequences. Been there, done that. Got the crutches.

If you've ever found yourself doing something really stupid on the road due to overly aggressive behavior, welcome to the club. If you're still doing it, sooner or later it will catch up to you. To change it (which benefits our health, our relationships, and our jobs) we must change how we think, feel, and act. But how?

There's an old riddle—what did the Zen Master say to the hot dog vendor? "Make me one with everything." So after getting the hot dog, he gives the vendor a $20 bill. The vendor puts it in his pocket and turns to the next customer. The Zen Master asks, "What about my change?!" The vendor answers, "Change must come from within."

Change is hard. Some folks manage to change by themselves—this is called "pulling yourself up by your own bootstraps." For many people, though, changing requires therapy.

There's a psychotherapy technique called cognitive behavioral therapy (CBT). The central concept involves understanding that *what you think* about a situation affects *what you feel*, and *what you feel* affects *how you act*. But what's most important, you can learn to control your reactions, which affects your feelings and behavior. CBT teaches you how you can choose your reaction in a given situation. An explanation of how this works is at an excellent website, www.cognitivetherapy.com. Here's their example of how thoughts influence emotions and actions.

Imagine your friend is meeting you for dinner, and it's an hour after she was supposed to arrive. Here are several scenarios illustrating how *what you think* affects *what you feel,* and *what you feel* affects *what you do.*

Scenario 1: You *think:* Maybe she had an accident. You *feel:* anxious or worried. You *do:* Call hospitals/ERs to find out if she's there.

Scenario 2: You *think:* She didn't even call to let me know she'd be late! You *feel:* angry, irritated. You *do:* Act cold or angry when she arrives.

Scenario 3: You *think:* I don't much care if folks are on time or not. You *feel:* indifferent. You *do:* Nothing special.

Scenario 4: You *think:* Great! I needed a little time to finish a project. You *feel:* Relieved. You *do:* Finish the project, and feel content and proud.

Of course, there are lots of different responses to the same scenario. But this shows how we respond is a learned behavior. And if we learn one behavior, we can learn another. That's what "therapy" is about—learning. And it's tough.

Personally, I've found it challenging to change my behaviors, despite the known benefits. Out here on the Left Coast, learning to change is called "personal growth" and it takes a long time to see results. Recently, though, I got this e-mail that is a good parable for the "growth" process.

An elderly Cherokee was teaching his grandchildren about life.

He said to them, "A fight is going on inside me, it is a terrible fight and it is between two wolves. One wolf is evil . . . he is fear, anger, envy, sorrow, regret, greed, arrogance, self-pity, guilt, resentment, inferiority, lies, false pride, aggressiveness, superiority, and ego."

"The other is good . . . he is joy, peace, love, hope, sharing, serenity, humility, kindness, benevolence, friendship, empathy, generosity, truth, and compassion. And the same fight is going on inside you and every other person, too."

The children thought about it for a minute, and then one child asked, "Which wolf will win?"

The old Cherokee answered, "The one you feed."

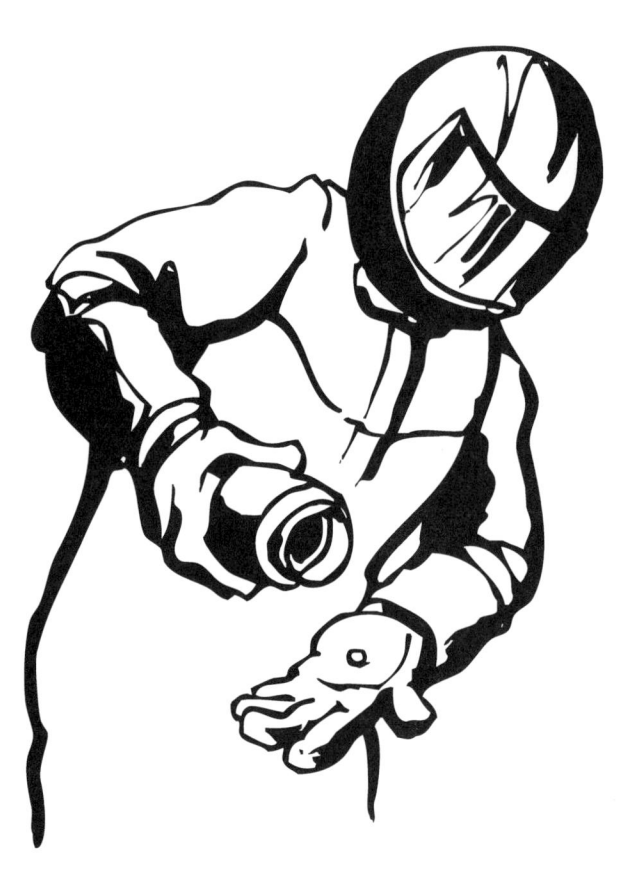

Hearts

One in four Americans who die each year drop dead from sudden cardiac death (SCD). That's one in four of *all deaths,* including accidents, injuries, crime, fires, cancer, infections, and all illnesses. That's the same odds as flipping a coin "heads" twice in a row. Many people who die from sudden cardiac death (SCD) have no heart disease history.

Dropping dead is a bad way to find out you've got a heart problem. It limits your options. You're much better off finding out in advance. If you've never had your cholesterol tested, especially with a family history of stroke or heart attacks, get it checked. If it's up, get it down! Even if you have normal cholesterol, you still might be at risk—half the people who drop dead have normal cholesterol.

Most people who die from SCD have one or more of these risk factors—high cholesterol, high blood pressure, diabetes, smoking, physical inactivity, obesity, and/or family history of cardiovascular disease (stroke or heart attack). Heart attacks often occur during exertion or strong emotion, but they can happen anytime, including during sleep. If this occurs, you wake up dead.

You can have a heart attack and not know it. Diagnosing one, even in an emergency room, can be difficult without specific blood tests. An electrocardiogram (EKG) can help, but a normal EKG does not rule out a myocardial infarction (AKA heart attack).

Classic symptoms include chest pain, shortness of breath, nausea, anxiety, sweating, and pain going down the left arm or up into the jaw. However, not all of these symptoms are present in every heart attack. Older people have fewer symptoms, or can have symptoms that aren't typical. But if you've got some or all of these, and might be having an MI, here's what to do.

First, Call an Ambulance.

Do not drive yourself to the ER, or have a friend or family member drive you. Remember that many people drop dead during the first hour after a heart attack, and others pass out from a bad heart rhythm. This is dangerous if you're driving or having someone drive you. While in an ambulance, EMS personnel can do CPR, and usually ACLS (Cardio Pulmonary Resuscitation and Advanced Cardiac Life Support) and your heart rhythm will be monitored.

After Calling EMS, You Should Chew an Aspirin.

That's right. Chew it, and then wash it down with water. Aspirin helps prevent the clot in your coronary artery that is causing the heart attack from growing and doing more damage. Blood clots usually cause heart attacks, not arteries filled with cholesterol, though cholesterol is often involved. *Remember, it must be an aspirin, not Tylenol, ibuprofen (Motrin, Advil) or other analgesic.*

Cholesterol (called "plaque") can accumulate under the lining of your coronary arteries, which then narrows. Lack of blood flow to an area of heart muscle may produce angina (chest pain). Since plaque is soft and unstable, the lining over it moves with each heartbeat and may eventually tear. High blood pressure makes this more likely. If the lining tears, the clotting elements in the blood (the platelets) start clotting to patch the hole. Sometimes, the clot that results can fill the whole artery. This cuts off blood supply to the heart muscle that artery feeds.

Clots can often be dissolved with "clot busting" drugs, restoring blood flow to your heart. To be effective, these must be used soon after the heart attack starts, which is another reason to use an ambulance to get to the ER—your car doesn't have flashing lights and a siren. It's also possible to open your clogged artery with a small balloon inserted into the coronary artery—an angioplasty.

After treatment, you'll be admitted to a CCU (coronary care unit) to monitor your heart rhythm and blood pressure. Problems, including sudden, potentially fatal rhythm changes, can be treated immediately in a CCU.

There are things you can do to avoid the above scenario. One of the easiest is to take a coated, 81 mg baby aspirin every day if you're a man over 40 who's diabetic, or has other increased risk factors, such as high cholesterol. Aspirin makes the platelets less sticky, which limits the size of a clot in a coronary. Of course, if you're on a medication like Coumadin (warfarin) or other blood-thinning medication already, this advice isn't for you. And if you've got an ulcer or other problems, or if bleeding is a health issue, ask your doctor.

Fish oil is another way to reduce your risk of SCD, since its omega-3 fatty acids not only make platelets less sticky, they help stabilize heart rhythms. Fish like wild salmon are high in omega-3—farmed salmon have less. Even canned albacore tuna has omega-3, but only if packed in water, not oil. Remember that pregnant women and children should minimize mercury intake, which is found in some fish.

Cholesterol: Nowadays, control is usually easy. Dieting is helpful, and statin medications like Lipitor®, Zocor®, Pravachol® and Vytorin® are very effective. Not only do they lower cholesterol, they make the coronary arteries' lining tougher and less likely to tear. I put all patients at high risk for coronary artery disease (including all diabetics) on statins. And statins can be combined with stanols like Benecol®, Cholestoff, and other brands to produce even more cholesterol lowering.

Blood pressure: Control is very important, and limits of acceptable BP have recently been lowered—130/85 for most folks, and 130/80 for diabetics. All diabetics should be on an ACE inhibitor drug like Capoten®, Vasotec®, or Zestril®, or on an angiotensin 2 receptor blocker like Cozaar® or Avapro®. Non-diabetics usually do well on a beta-blocker like Tenormin®, Inderal®, or Toprol®, and/or a diuretic like hydrochlorthiazide.

Smoking: It's tough to change, though you can reduce your risk to that of a non-smoker ten years after you quit. I've had the best results using a Nicotrol® Inhaler—a great product. It provides all the benefits and pleasure of nicotine without the carcinogens and carbon monoxide of smoking. And you can do it in a restaurant, airplane, or movie theater.

Physical inactivity: This can be a tough risk factor to change for folks short on time. It takes about an hour's walking seven days a week to change your metabolism and significantly lower your cardiac risk. Running, biking, or swimming for less time gives you the same benefit, but do something *every day*.

Family history: Next time, pick healthier ancestors.

And if you don't want to modify your risk factors, just remember the old saying,

"Don't worry about your heart. It's got a lifetime warranty."

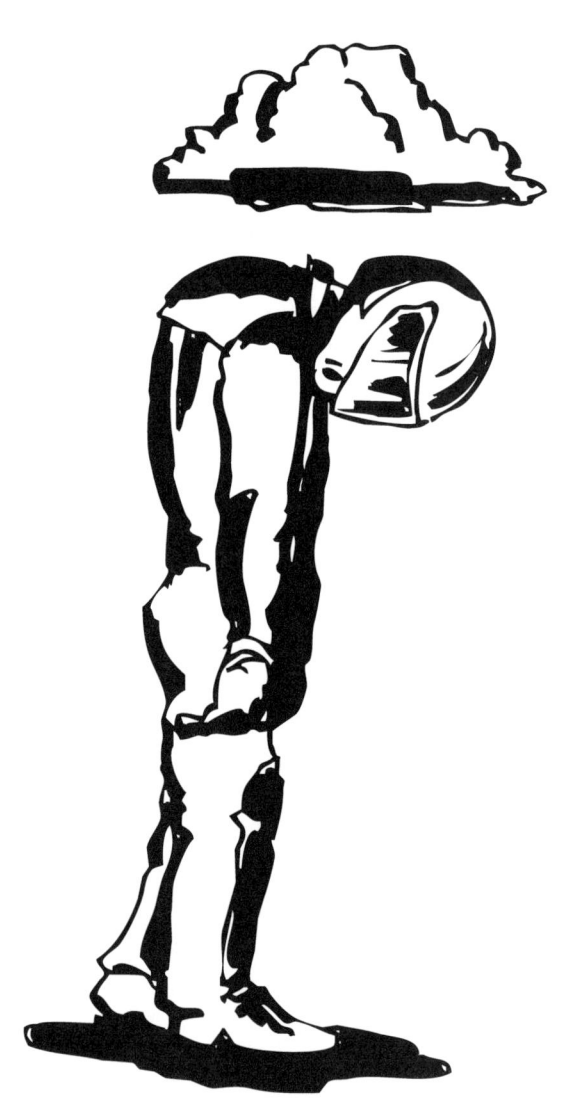

Depression

Recently I was talking to a very experienced rider. He noticed he'd been taking more risks than usual, which was strange, considering he's one of the most safety-oriented people I know. I asked if there was a possibility he might be depressed, since I've known folks to have less of a sense of self-preservation when they're feeling down on themselves. After consideration and further discussion, we agreed that might be the problem.

Depression is extremely common. It's the leading cause of disability in the U.S., and affects about 1 in 10 people every year. Over 40, that figure is 1 in 5. Not only does it take the joy out of a person's motorcycling (and out of everything else in their life), it often has bad effects on that person's family, friends, and the folks he works with. It's even sometimes fatal, though it's usually easy to treat. Worse, many folks don't admit or even know they're depressed, and don't get any help.

Here's a depression quiz. If you answer the first two questions yes, plus a few of the others, talk to your primary care doc about the possibility of depression. Take this list with you.

Both of these:
- I am really sad most of the time.
- I don't enjoy doing the things I've always enjoyed doing.

Plus a few of these:
- I don't sleep well at night and am very restless.
- I am always tired. I find it hard to get out of bed.
- I don't feel like eating much.
- I feel like eating all the time.
- I have lots of aches and pains that don't go away.
- I have little to no sexual energy.
- I find it hard to focus and am becoming very forgetful.
- I am mad at everybody and everything.
- I feel upset and fearful, but can't figure out why.
- I don't feel like talking to people.

- I feel like there isn't much point to living, nothing good is going to happen to me.
- I don't like myself very much. I feel bad most of the time.
- I think about death a lot. I even think about how I might kill myself.

There are medical problems that can make folks feel depressed—low thyroid, for example. Your family doctor can tell the difference. One central finding in depression is not enjoying things that are usually fun (anhedonia).

Here's a site that has men describing how depression has affected them: tinyurl.com/ojvc. And here's some general info: tinyurl.com/pco7.

There are different varieties of depression. In major depression, there's at least two weeks of sad mood, loss of interest/ enjoyment of usually fun activities, as well as several of the symptoms on the above list. Depression causes problems with work, study, fun, sex drive, sleep, and eating. Folks who've had one episode of major depression are at higher risk to have another one.

Dysthymia is a milder form of depression. It doesn't usually cause disability by itself, but folks with dysthymia often have a chronic low mood, lack of energy, and sometimes episodes of major depression.

Another form of depression is bipolar disorder, which used to be called "manic-depressive" disorder. Folks with this problem alternate periods of depressed mood with periods of increased energy, little sleep, and (often) disordered thinking.

Recently, it's been shown that some people have a genetic predisposition for depression. There's a gene called the "serotonin transporter gene," which is found in two forms—a short version and a long version. Folks with one or two copies of the short version (you get your chromosomes from both your parents, and have two copies of most genes) are a lot more likely to get depressed in response to stress, illness, or other difficult situations. Folks with two copies of the long version tend not to suffer depression. (Please note that this gene test isn't widely available yet.)

You often hear about "serotonin" in relation to depression. Serotonin is a chemical that nerve cells use to communicate. The most common drugs used for depression are selective serotonin reuptake inhibitors (SSRIs) like Prozac®, Paxil®, etc., which are usually effective after a few weeks. Recent research has shown that growing new nerve cells in the part of the brain called the hippocampus is necessary for mice to recover from depression. Blocking this growth prevents SSRIs from working. This might explain why most folks don't benefit immediately from SSRIs—it takes several weeks to grow new cells.

Nerve cells outside the brain are also affected by serotonin, too. The gut has many nerve cells, which explains the temporary GI changes that are common in the first week of taking an SSRI. Some people get constipated, while others get a slight case of the runs. This goes away after a week or so. Other occasional side effects (headache, etc.) are mildly unpleasant and go away quickly, too.

One side effect common to many SSRIs is sexual dysfunction. Some people have difficulty climaxing. Others lose interest. And this side effect tends to last—it doesn't go away. Wellbutrin® (buproprion), though, doesn't cause this problem, and when given along with an SSRI may prevent or eliminate the problem.

Depression tends to respond well to both medications and to talk therapy, though talk therapy takes longer to start making much difference. When I put a patient on an SSRI, chances are very good that he'll/she'll feel much better in four to six weeks. It often takes six months to get the same good effects from talk therapy.

Using both medications and talk therapy is often very effective. Depression often causes lack of energy—people just don't feel like doing anything. When the meds kick in, they have an easier time dealing with their problems.

Contrary to what some folks think, SSRIs and other antidepressants are *not* tranquilizers—they don't make you into a zombie. Most folks are able to enjoy things again. Their appetites normalize, they're sleeping better, and they start to get out and do things and have fun doing them.

And that's what life's all about.

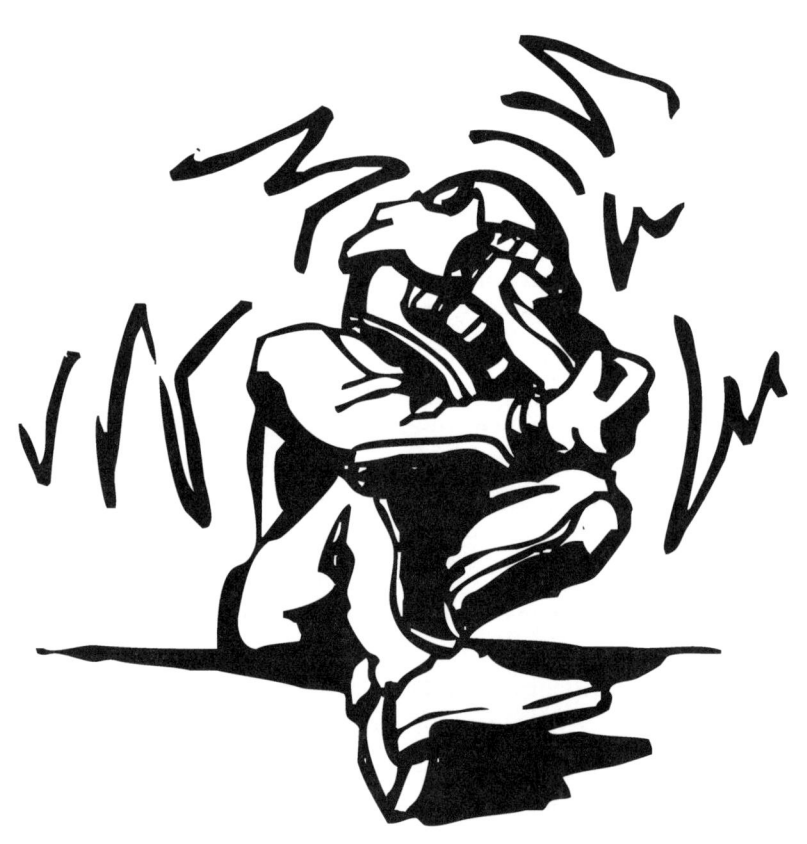

Post-Traumatic Stress Disorder

Ever had an accident? Afterward, did you find yourself feeling jumpy, thinking about the accident all the time, not sleeping, getting excessively nervous when riding, or avoiding riding (or a particular kind of riding) altogether? If so, you may have post-traumatic stress disorder (PTSD).

For 25 percent of men and 13 percent of women, accidents are the most psychologically traumatic event in their lives. Mental health problems after severe emotional trauma can include post-traumatic stress disorder, major depression, and anxiety issues. PTSD is the most common of these problems, accounting for about 60 percent of the mental problems people have after accidents. About one in 10 people who have an accident will develop PTSD.

Factors that increase the likelihood of developing PTSD after an accident include the amount of injury suffered, as well as the fear generated by the accident. Since motorcyclists have increased vulnerability in an accident, they're at higher risk for developing PTSD (i.e., more likely to be injured in an accident than a car driver). If the accident results in a dramatic change of lifestyle (like being unable to ride anymore) the risk of PTSD increases. This is another reason why it's important to get back on the bike—continuing a previous lifestyle can decrease your risk of emotional problems.

How does somebody know if they've got PTSD? To have actual PTSD requires a number of factors. First, there must be a "stressor event." The event has to involve actual or threatened injury or death, and the person undergoing the event has to experience intense fear, helplessness, or horror at that time. Having a strong emotional reaction at or around the time of the event is an essential element of PTSD. It's been theorized that chemical changes in your brain associated with the stress play an essential element in the development of the problem.

After the event, the person must suffer what's called "intrusive recollections." These may persist for decades or an entire lifetime. They can occur during the daytime, or as nightmares, or as a re-enactment called a "PTSD flashback." Things that remind the person of the event may also cause similar reactions. If you had a bad accident while riding in the rain, for example, wet roads may cause you to experience a disproportionate sense of anxiety if you have PTSD.

Another element of PTSD is called the avoidant/numbing reaction. A person with PTSD will try to avoid any kind of activity or stimulus that might cause him to be reminded of the event. If someone was injured very badly while doing wheelies, for example, they might be more likely to avoid that activity in the future. (Some people might prefer to call this "evolution in action.") Another kind of avoidant behavior is called "psychic numbing," in which people with PTSD try to avoid strong emotions that they might associate with the accident event. This may cause them to try to avoid emotions altogether, which often makes it difficult for them to have meaningful interpersonal relationships.

PTSD victims also have symptoms called hyperarousal. Insomnia and irritability are common examples of this, but even more characteristic of PTSD are the hypervigilance and excessive startle reflexes. People with PTSD can be excessively jumpy—a loud noise may set them off. A good way to describe them would be "twitchy" (think of "Tweek" in South Park).

To qualify as real PTSD, the symptoms must last for at least a month, and cause problems at work, at home, or in other aspects of life. But it's also possible that PTSD may not surface for years. Sometimes, the victim doesn't have symptoms until he experiences something that resembles the initial event. For example, if someone had a bad accident and didn't have problems afterward, a second accident might cause full-blown PTSD.

How do you prevent PTSD? Well, avoiding accidents is a good idea, as is avoiding other traumatic situations. Unfortunately, life doesn't give us that choice. People whose coping skills and social support networks are good before the event tend to do better afterward. Early treatment after the event may help prevent PTSD, so if you have PTSD symptoms after a traumatic event, tell your doctor.

What's the best treatment for PTSD? A number of different treatments have been shown to be successful, though some cases may be resistant to therapy. First is cognitive behavioral therapy (CBT), which is based on the theory that it's our thoughts that cause our emotional reactions, not external events. This makes sense, since the same event can cause different reactions in different people. The difference is what you think about the event. Waking up to find a tarantula on your pillow would be extremely stressful for most people. However, a person who had a pet tarantula might only be mildly annoyed that it had gotten out of its cage. CBT can do a number of other things. These include specific techniques for dealing with anxiety, such as breath training, how to deal with negative thoughts, managing anger, getting ready to deal with stress reactions, dealing with the urge to drink or use drugs to control trauma symptoms, and rebuilding social skills.

Medications are often used for PTSD. Though Zoloft® and Paxil® are approved, other SSRIs, such as Celexa®, Lexapro®, and Prozac®, are also helpful. Other medications that reduce anxiety such as Valium®, Ativan®, and Xanax® are sometimes used, but long-term use of these kinds of tranquilizers occasionally leads to problems. Xanax® in particular is very habit-forming, and sudden discontinuation can cause a panic attack.

Group therapy has been shown to be very good for treating PTSD. It allows people to share experiences in a safe and supportive environment. Other therapies include desensitization, in which people are exposed to stressors in a controlled fashion, and Eye Movement Desensitization and Reprocessing (EMDR), though this technique is relatively new and not completely accepted. The take-home message is this. Don't ignore feelings of anxiety, insomnia, jumpiness, or intrusive thoughts after a traumatic episode. Though the symptoms may improve by themselves, seeing a professional may prevent many years of problems.

Fitness for Riding

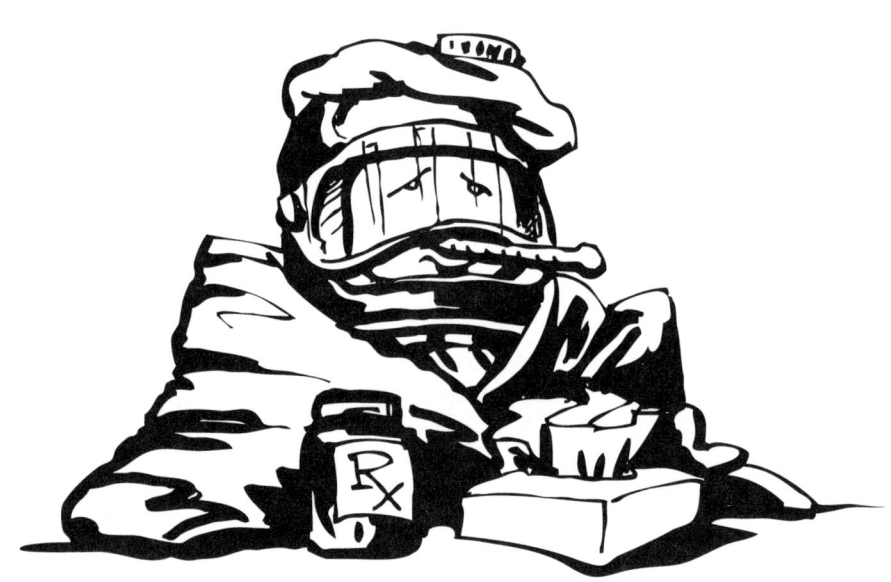

The Common Cold:
Nothing to Sneeze At

Have you ever sneezed inside your face shield? It's not pretty. And since you always close your eyes while sneezing, colds impact safety, too. (I use the word "impact" deliberately). Though there's no cure for the common cold, an "ounce of prevention" helps. One reason there's no cure is that over a hundred different viruses cause colds, with the rhinovirus family (nose viruses) responsible for half. And even if a vaccine were developed against one virus, the rest could still infect you.

When cold viruses enter the cells in your nose, they hijack their production systems and start making new viruses. This "incubation period" takes 10 to 12 hours. After that, your nose makes lots of new cold viruses, and you start having symptoms. You'll get worse for a day or so, until your body makes antibodies against that cold virus.

The best and easiest way to keep from catching a cold is removing the viruses from your hands before you infect yourself, which only takes soap and water. Another technique is using an alcohol-containing gel, like Purell. Though soap and water works better, using gels can reduce germ counts.

The greatest public health advance in history was the public acceptance of hand washing to remove germs. Amazingly, it wasn't until 1867 that Joseph Lister came up with the idea of sterilizing surgical instruments after they were used on sick patients, and it wasn't until the beginning of the twentieth century that rubber gloves were routinely used in surgery.

If prevention fails, what next? You might say "I'll just take some Contac® or Theraflu® or Actifed®" Don't. These products contain antihistamines and decongestants, which dry you out. If you feel like a Vesuvius of snot, being dried out sounds good, but here's why it's such a bad idea. The total surface area of all the tiny air sacs in your lungs is about twice the size of a tennis court. Imagine how fast moisture evaporates from that size area! It's important to keep your lungs moist, since their natural secretions become hard and sticky when dry (think of your nose in the desert). These hard, dry secretions (which I call "phlegm boogers") then block your bronchial passages, which can cause bronchitis and sometimes pneumonia. Drying agents like antihistamine/decongestant combos are particularly hazardous for folks who have asthma, or who have a tendency for colds that "go to their chest."

So, what do you do when your nose goes on strike? (No, not "picket," dummy!) As long as you don't have high blood pressure or a heart condition, it's usually safe to use decongestant pills and/or nose spray for a short time. I recommend the 12-hour sprays that have oxymetazoline 0.05 percent (Afrin®) as the active ingredient. But don't use it for more than a week—the rebound congestion gets many people hooked.

Another helpful medicine is pseudoephedrine (Sudafed®), which is available in tablet and capsule form. I like the 30mg tablets, since it's easier to adjust the dose than it is with the 12-hour timed-release capsule. Be careful that whatever you get has *only* pseudoephedrine in it. There's a Sudafed® brand cold medicine that also has antihistamines.

Although decongestant nose sprays and decongestant pills do dry you out, they have the big advantage of not causing drowsiness. In fact, many folks feel a little jittery on decongestants, which can cause problems sleeping. Luckily, taking 50mg of diphenhydramine (Benadryl®) at bedtime will help both a runny nose, a cough, and your sleep, since antihistamines (particularly the older, first-generation ones) help tire you out, too.

One product I've found very helpful for a stuffy nose is Breathe Right® nasal strips. They pull the nose open wider and work very well. You may have seen athletes wearing them—they improve airflow a lot. It's important to wash the nose with soap and water first to remove skin oils, and to position it correctly. They make it much easier to sleep with nasal congestion, and you don't wake up dopey, or with a dried-out sore throat.

You might be tempted to take antihistamines while riding. This is a bad idea. Did you know that the most common drugs found in the bloodstream of pilots who've crashed are antihistamines? In such cases, antihistamines are more common than alcohol, sedatives, or narcotics, and they're also linked to motor vehicle accidents and workplace injuries. They're dangerous to take while driving, especially the older antihistamines like Benadryl®, Chlortrimeton®, and those found in the OTC cold medications mentioned above.

Newer drugs that are called "non-sedating" such as Claritin®, Clarinex®, Allegra®, and Zyrtec® are less effective at helping a runny nose, and are less sedating than older antihistamines. They still may increase your crash risk, though. In the studies I've seen, Zyrtec® is a little sedating; Claritin® and Clarinex® are less, and Allegra® doesn't have much, if any, sedating effect.

Remember, it only takes from 1 to 30 virus particles to transmit an infection—they're incredibly contagious. Doorknobs, cups or glasses, pencils, faucets, telephones, toilet handles—all these can transmit live viruses. But most viruses don't penetrate intact skin. They get in your system when you touch your eyes, nose, mouth, or lips, which most people do every four minutes or so. Think of it this way: When you touch your face or eat something, it's exactly as if you licked everything you touched since last washing your hands. Airborne spread from sneezing and coughing is another source of contagion; but don't skip washing.

Of course, if you're in a confined space (like an airline cabin) your risk of catching somebody's cold is higher than if you're outside. Whenever I fly, I always wear a paper dust mask (like the ones used for sanding) to keep floating mucus droplets out. My wife prefers to use a scarf as a bandanna for the same purpose. Of course, if you decide to use the bandanna method, don't put it on until *after* you're seated on the aircraft . . .

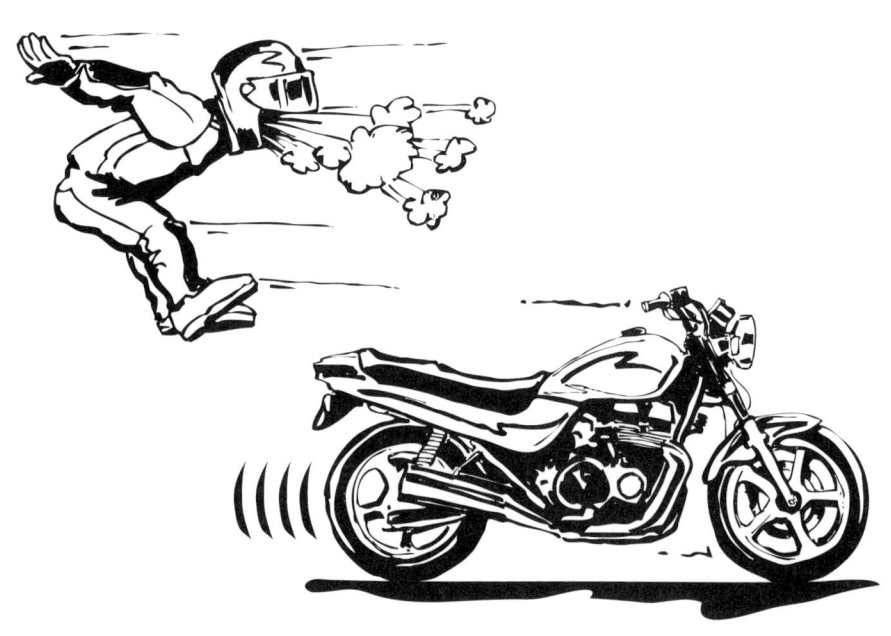

Allergies

Allergies are often worse certain times of the year. Spring is bad, since plants bloom, releasing pollens. If you're allergic, your body reacts to these pollens and to other allergens (things you're allergic to) as if they're invading organisms. It tries to kill them. Mold releases spores when humidity rises, triggering allergies in people with mold allergies when it rains or gets damp.

Allergies can be confused with an upper respiratory infection, like a cold. Though symptoms may be similar at first, colds eventually involve more systems than just your nose. They'll usually cause fever, muscle aches, and sometimes nausea, vomiting, and/or diarrhea. Allergies won't.

Colds may resemble allergies since the body's defense mechanisms against cold viruses and allergens are similar. Your nose gets stuffy and runny, you sneeze, and sometimes you cough. This is how your body tries to trap and eliminate invaders, which may be bacteria, virus, or allergens.

Treatments for allergies vary. Most work by convincing your body not to fight so hard, or by blocking some of your body's defense mechanisms.

Histamine is a substance that's central in your body's response to a perceived threat. It's released by mast cells after your body "recognizes" enemies. It makes blood vessels leak a little, in order to get some of your body's defense mechanisms out into the tissue where the "problem" is. When this happens in your nose, after you breathe in an allergen, it causes the nasal tissue to swell and get more moist. The resulting stuffy, runny nose is part of the histamine response.

Antihistamines block this response, more or less, and may help stop the runny nose and itchy eyes typical of many allergies. The problem is that the antihistamines available without prescription impair your functioning even if you don't feel sleepy. What's more, you're more likely to fall asleep with antihistamines on board.

Case in point: Benadryl® (diphenhydramine), a strong, over-the-counter (OTC) antihistamine, is also sold as Sominex®, a sleeping pill. Most of the cold and cough remedies, like Actifed®, Dimetapp®, Theraflu®, and Nyquil®, also have sedating antihistamines. Don't take them and ride or drive.

As I mentioned before, the newer class of "non-sedating" antihistamines are less sedating than the older ones, but also not as powerful as older antihistamines. Zyrtec (cetirizine) is the strongest antihistamine, but does cause some drowsiness in some people. I'd be a little leery of taking it while riding. Allegra® is the least sedating antihistamine available.

If you get allergies that mostly affect your nose, the steroid nasal sprays are a very good choice. They work by stabilizing the cells that cause the release of histamine. In other words, they convince your nose not to worry about the allergens floating by. Flonase® (fluticasone), Beconase® (beclomethasone), and Nasonex® (mometasone) are examples of this class of meds, and fluticasone is now available as a generic, which is cheaper. They only need to be used once a day, and have no systemic effects. After using this kind of medication for a few days, most folks feel like their nose moved to the New Mexico desert—their allergies disappear.

Decongestants, like Sudafed® (pseudoephedrine), are also popular for allergies, but they should be used with caution. They constrict blood vessels inside your nose, drying it out. When your nose is running, "drying it out" sounds good, but since a dry nose can't moisturize the air going to your lungs, your lungs get dried out, too. Then, the mucus lining the lungs' airways gets hard and sticky, and stays there inside your bronchial tubes. Not only does this cause irritation that can trigger asthma, but it can also cause some people who've never known they had asthma to start wheezing. It can also cause bronchitis or pneumonia. If you take decongestants, be sure to drink enough liquids so your urine is almost clear.

There's another class of medications, called "mast cell stabilizers," that is very useful for some kinds of allergies. If used before you're exposed, it can prevent you from reacting—for example, you might use a mast cell stabilizer before visiting a friend with a cat, or riding through an area you know will have a lot of pollen.

Nasalcrom® (cromolyn) is available for use in the nose, and similar medications can be used in the eyes and lungs. They have very few side effects and are worth a try. Their downside is that they're only effective in about half the folks who use them—but those people often get dramatic results.

Not all allergies affect the nose and/or lungs. Many people get red, itchy, watery eyes from allergies. There are antihistamine eye drops available without prescription that can be helpful, but they shouldn't be used for more than a few days. If used too long, you may get a "rebound effect," with worsening of your symptoms. Prescription antihistamine eye drops are useful, too, but like the OTC drops, many need to be used, often—sometimes four times a day. There are "mast cell stabilizer" eye drops available, too.

Acular® is another very useful eye medication—it often works like magic. It's a non-steroidal anti-inflammatory, and works very quickly, often stopping all symptoms within five minutes. Note that if you wear soft contact lenses, you need to leave them out for five minutes after putting the drops in. If your eyes bother you a lot during allergy season, and an antihistamine or mast cell stabilizer doesn't do the trick, ask your doc about Acular®.

The take-home message here is that allergies are more serious than just a little stuffy nose. They can affect your lungs, your sinuses, and they can even trigger an asthma attack. So remember, allergies are nothing to sneeze at.

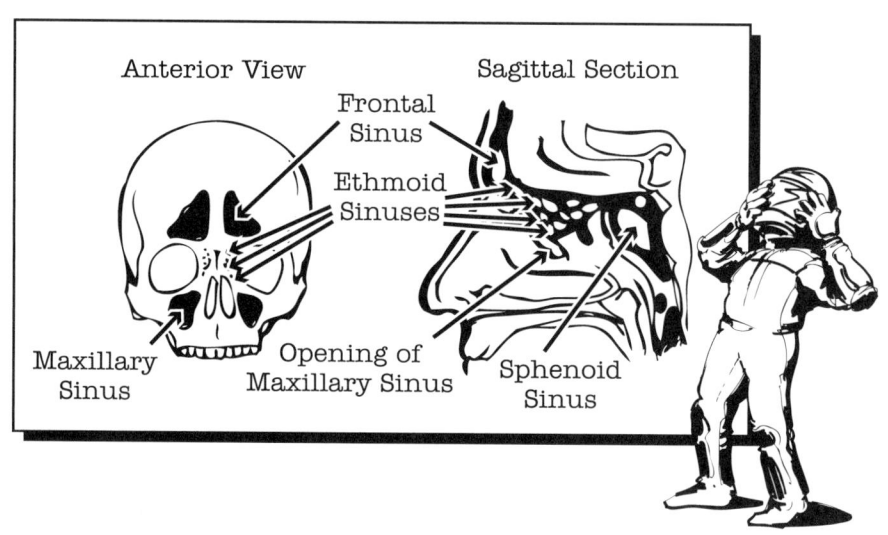

Anterior View   Sagittal Section

Frontal
Sinus

Ethmoid
Sinuses

Maxillary
Sinus

Opening of
Maxillary Sinus

Sphenoid
Sinus

Sinuses

You need a sinus like you need a hole in the head. In fact, that's what a sinus is. Sinuses make the skull lighter; help your voice resonate; and provide a "crumple zone" to help protect your brain when your face hits something (or something hits you) very hard. You've got sinuses in your cheeks, behind the bridge of your nose, and in your forehead. If you put both hands flat over your face, they'll cover your sinuses.

Sinuses are lined with the same kind of mucus producing membrane that lines your nose and lungs. This "ciliated mucus membrane" is designed to catch dust and germs, like flypaper, and then sweep the mucus to the sinus opening. All your sinuses have a small opening emptying into your nasal cavity.

People's sinus openings vary in size. Those folks with long, narrow faces tend to have more sinus problems—people with the "Prince Charles" type of face. People who look like Nanook the Eskimo don't get blocked sinuses as often.

Anything that makes your nose run causes your sinuses to produce more mucus, too. Allergies can do it, as can colds or exposure to irritants. If the sinuses can't empty as fast as the mucus is made, you've got a problem.

Two factors really affect the sinuses' ability to drain—cigarette smoke and dryness. The nicotine in the tobacco paralyzes the cells that sweep out the dust and germ-laden mucus. Dryness makes the mucus much harder and stickier. If you've ever spent time outside in a hot, dry, dusty place, you know how the mucus in your nose gets hard. Your sinuses are designed to move moist, liquid mucus, not rocks.

Things get worse quickly when the opening to the sinus gets blocked by one of these chunks of dried mucus. The cells that produce the mucus keep producing it, even though the sinus isn't draining normally. The additional mucus increases the pressure in the sinus, and this pressure causes pain. And once you've got a pool of stagnant mucus in one of your sinuses, it's ripe for infection. There's nothing more appetizing to a germ than a pool of stagnant mucus. Yum!

Once a sinus is infected, the real trouble starts. High pressure in the sinus impairs the blood flow, and the body can't get white blood cells into the area to fight the infection. The germs then grow unopposed, and you can find yourself with a very serious condition. People can die from bad sinus infections that don't get treated properly.

An infected sinus hurts. The skin over the sinus may be tender, warm or red; there's usually green drainage, and you may have a fever. This is a medical emergency. When a sinus gets a bacterial infection, antibiotics can save your life. See your doctor without delay.

Typically, I'll prescribe amoxicillin for a first sinus infection. If it's a recurrent one, or if the person's at higher risk because of other conditions, I'll often use Augmentin® or Levaquin®. I'll almost always prescribe a nasal steroid spray, too, since they've been shown to help an infection by shrinking inflamed tissues and promoting drainage.

Two things are necessary to treat sinus infections—drain the sinus and kill the germs. Of the two, drainage is the most important. Remember the dried mucus that can plug the sinus opening? This is contributing to the problem. To loosen it, drink lots of extra fluids (try to consume enough to make your urine clear) and get more moisture in the air you're breathing. Closing the doors and windows of your bathroom (with the fan off) while taking a hot shower can help; so can putting your face over a steaming hot pan of water with a towel over your head. If you can moisten the piece of dried mucus that's blocking the tiny sinus opening, you might make it slippery enough to slip out.

Other factors that contribute to blocking the sinuses include swollen mucus membranes. If your nose is stuffy and it's hard to breath, chances are the openings to your sinuses are swollen and it's hard for them to drain, too. One of the few times that I recommend decongestants like Sudafed® (pseudoephedrine) is when a sinus is blocked. If you do take them, take extra fluids! I also recommend a 12-hour nasal spray containing oxymetozaline (Afrin®

is the best known) to shrink swollen membranes and promote drainage.

It's important to use decongestant nasal sprays correctly. Don't use them for more than five days, or you'll get rebound congestion when stopping.

Once your nose is open, it would be a good time to breathe in the steam I mentioned earlier. Also, if one side of your face is more affected than the other, sleep with the bad side up. It's easier for a sinus to drain downhill. Also, many people find an ice pack is very effective at relieving the pain and pressure from a sinus infection.

Lastly, remember that tobacco smoke paralyzes your sinus linings, as well as your lungs. So if you've got a sinus problem, you need cigarettes like you need a hole in the head.

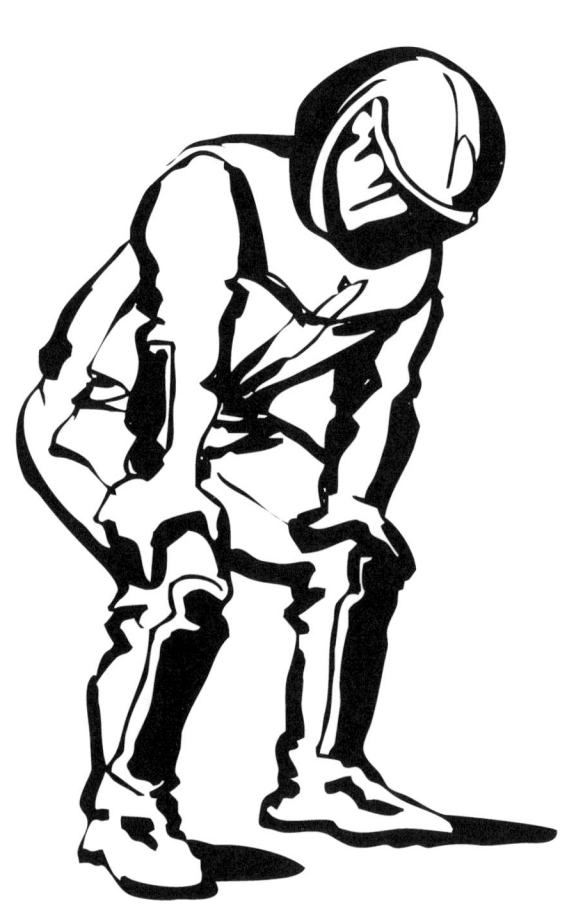

Asthma

"I don't have asthma!" is something I hear every week, all winter long. And every winter, I find dozens of folks with asthma who don't know they have it. And undiagnosed asthma is *never* treated correctly. Here's what typically happens.

The patient comes in complaining of a chest cold lasting a few weeks. They might have a dry cough, or perhaps they're bringing up a little clear phlegm. Often, there's a history of chest colds, commonly in the fall or winter. Another common story is somebody who first develops hay fever symptoms (itchy eyes, runny nose) and then starts coughing (allergies go with asthma). I'll ask them if they had asthma as a child; some say, "yes, but I outgrew it," or, "no, but I had chest colds a lot."

When I hear this, I think "asthmatic in denial," AKA Cleopatra syndrome (Cleopatra/denial? Oh, never mind).

What is asthma? It's just the tendency for bronchial tubes to constrict in response to things like allergies, exercise, cold, aspirin, irritation, or air pollution. Most people (including some doctors) think, "If you don't wheeze, you don't have asthma." This is wrong—there are millions of people who never wheeze, but still have asthma. There's also "cough variant asthma" that gives patients a dry cough, with no wheezing or shortness of breath. Congestive heart failure can cause wheezing, too, but "cardiac asthma" isn't asthma.

Patients with heartburn (AKA GERD: gastro-esophageal reflux disease) often get asthma that goes away when their reflux is treated. If someone has heartburn and a cough, daily heartburn treatment with something like Prilosec® a half-hour before breakfast often cures the cough, too.

If someone with childhood asthma still gets chest colds, they probably still have asthma (though smokers, frequent fliers, and parents of kids in day care get chest colds, too). Asthmatics' bronchial tubes are generally more sensitive for a lifetime.

Another variant of asthma is "exercise-induced" asthma. It's one of the most common forms in kids, and is often the reason some kids "don't like sports." Since it causes shortness of breath (with or without wheezing) upon exercise, kids with this condition often don't like to run or bike hard. If a kid complains he gets out of breath easily, don't just assume he or she's out of shape. Ask the doctor to check for exercise-induced asthma. When controlled, exercise-induced asthmatics can excel at sports. About 20 percent of US Winter Olympic athletes have had asthma, and asthmatics on the 1984 US Olympic teams won 41 medals (15 gold, 20 silver and 6 bronze).

The take-home message is that asthma can present you with nothing more than a mild memory problem; a dry, nagging cough (sometimes at night); occasional chest colds; or even just getting out of breath easily when exercising. "Not wheezing" isn't "not having asthma." If someone has even mild asthma symptoms, ask the doctor to check the peak flow (or another breathing test, like an FEV-1) before and 20 minutes after treatment with a bronchodilator like albuterol. If the breathing improves by 15 percent or so, treating the person for asthma is a good idea.

Asthma treatment has changed a lot in the last several years. In the past, bronchodilators like albuterol (Ventolin®, Proventil®) were the mainstays of asthma treatment. Now, many patients are on a long-acting bronchodilator like Foradil® or Serevent® in addition to an anti-inflammatory. For exercise-induced asthma, Serevent® alone, before exercise, is a very good treatment.

Folks getting symptoms more than a couple of times a week should all be on anti-inflammatories like an inhaled steroid, such as Pulmicort®, Beclovent®, Vanceril®, Azmacort®, Flovent®, or Aerobid®. These prevent the inflammation that triggers asthma. Other anti-inflammatories are "leukotriene inhibitor" pills (Singulair®, Accolate®, and Zyflo®), which are used for both asthma and for allergies. I don't use them as first-line treatment, but some patients can benefit a lot.

Many people get nervous at the mention of the word "steroid," especially in Marin County, where I practice. Actually, using inhaled steroids for asthma is much safer and healthier than not using them, since more people die now from asthma than in the past. Inhaled steroids typically only act on the lungs, though oral steroids, like prednisone, are sometimes given for severe asthma. Though systemic (oral) steroids can cause problems over the long run, brief use for an asthma flare-up can be lifesaving. And since asthma can lead to emphysema, AKA chronic obstructive lung disease (which is incurable) under-treating asthma is harmful. In fact, the Sanskrit word for life, soul, and breath are all the same—Atman.

Since about two-thirds of asthmatics also have nasal allergies, most of my asthmatics use nasal steroids (Beconase®, Flonase®, Rhinocort®, Nasacort®, Nasonex®, Nasalide®, and Vancenase®) when their allergies act up. A runny nose usually runs down the throat, and can irritate the lungs, triggering asthma. As I've said before, "allergies are nothing to sneeze at." This is extra important for asthmatics.

Another problem for some asthmatics is aspirin. Not only can it trigger asthma, but it also can lead to growths inside the nose called "nasal polyps." If you're an asthmatic and your nose is always stuffy you should get checked for this, too.

Breathing—It's a good thing.

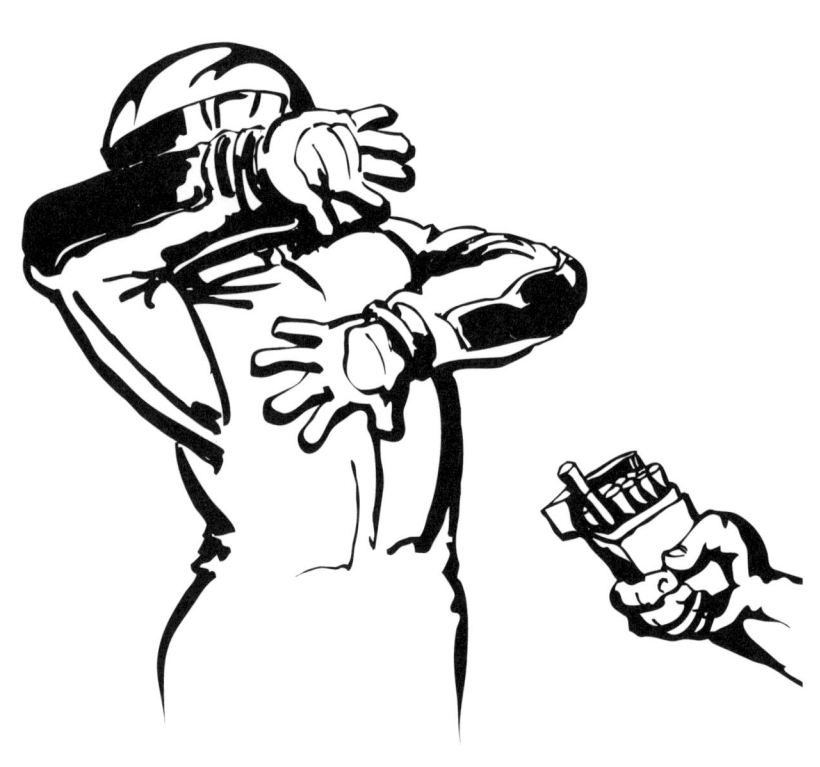

Smoking: Don't Say, "I'll Never Smoke Again"

Nicotine's a wonderful drug. It helps you relax, aids digestion, and improves your mood. You can concentrate better. It's an immediate mild antidepressant (unlike prescription anti-depressants, which take weeks to kick in). And it gives you something to do with your hands. These good effects are why folks keep smoking despite the 50 percent chance of dying or becoming disabled from it.

Unfortunately, nicotine is also addictive and lethal. Sooner or later, though, you probably get tired of not being in control of your life. You find yourself standing in the rain outside a building holding a newspaper over your head getting a nicotine hit. Or you get jittery after 45 minutes in a movie, and go outside and miss a crucial plot point. Or you're in a restaurant that doesn't allow smoking, and can't wait to get outside. Or you have to stop for a smoke after only 60 or 70 miles, which annoys you (and your riding companions).

So you've been thinking of quitting—you've even tried to quit before. Don't get discouraged if you've fallen off the wagon—it's just like riding a bike. Get back on and try again. Most smokers quit five or six times before they're ultimately successful.

Smoking is both a physical addiction and a psychological habit. Each reinforces the other. The physical addiction kicks in after 45 minutes without a smoke, as nicotine levels fall. The psychological habit part kicks in at a gas stop after a long ride, or after a meal, or when working on the computer—times you're used to smoking. Both of these aspects back each other up. Nicotine withdrawal and certain situations are cues to smoke. And since smoking is pleasurable, you keep doing it.

Despite nicotine's benefits, many smokers want to quit. But they still see images that prod them to smoke again—billboards, in-store advertising, people in movies and on TV. I once had a patient put it this way:

"Doc, cigarettes have been my friend for years and years. They're like a faithful dog—always there when I need 'em, and a constant source of comfort. You're asking me to get rid of that dog. And not only that, everywhere I go I see my dog lookin' at me from signs and I see folks with him on TV, and I can have him back for a few bucks. That makes it really hard for me to stop smoking."

He's right. Quitting smoking is one of the toughest things to do. I've known people who've managed to beat heroin or alcohol addiction, who still aren't able to quit nicotine. Most folks who do quit aren't successful until the sixth or seventh time. Here's why it's so hard.

When you smoke, you get the nicotine into your brain almost instantly. If you swallow a pill, it'll usually take at least 10 or 15 minutes before it gets into your brain. If you get an injection in a muscle, it takes a minute or so to hit. Getting medication intravenously—that is, shooting it into a vein—takes 10 or 15 seconds to make it to your brain.

But when you smoke something like nicotine or crack cocaine, the drug only has to go through the lining of the lungs' alveoli (air sacs) into the blood in your lungs. This is really quick, since the alveolar walls are only one cell thick, and have an area of about twice that of a tennis court. The cup or so of blood that's in your lungs is spread out over this area, so absorption is nearly instantaneous.

The next heartbeat usually occurs less than a second later. It moves the blood from your lungs through your heart and pumps it toward your body and your brain. A heartbeat later and the drug is affecting your central nervous system. Since you feel its action so quickly, you get immediate reinforcement. The speed of its action also lets you adjust the level of the drug precisely, so you get just the effect you want. These factors make nicotine addiction much harder to break.

Some folks stop cold turkey. This is possible, but it takes a lot of will power (or more properly, *won't* power). The advantages are that it's fast and you feel better sooner. Most folks who quit feel better in just a day or two, since they lose the carbon monoxide that's in their blood, preventing it from carrying all the oxygen that it can.

Up to 20 percent of the hemoglobin in a smoker's blood (that is, the red part of the blood that carries the oxygen) has carbon monoxide stuck tightly to it, forming carboxyhemoglobin. Since the CO (carbon monoxide) sticks tighter than oxygen, it can take a day or two to get unstuck after you quit. When this happens, it's like getting a blood transfusion—you get more energy, more stamina, and are able to concentrate better.

The brain uses more oxygen than other organs, and so the relative lack of oxygen caused by carboxyhemoglobin causes some impairment of memory and thinking. Many people report that they stop forgetting things so much after their brain starts to get more oxygen—in other words, they don't have as many "senior moments" (which are technically termed "brain farts"). More blood gets to your muscles, too. I've had patients tell me they can walk up a hill without getting out of breath that they couldn't have a week earlier.

Since stopping smoking is so hard, but has so many health benefits, there are many programs all over the country to help folks quit. Some are commercial ones like Smokenders, which has been around for 34 years. The fact they're still in business speaks well of their methods. If they didn't work, they wouldn't still be here. Many health organizations either sponsor or have information about programs. Kaiser Permanente offers stop smoking classes that are effective, and you can contact your local American Heart Association, the American Lung Association, and of course the American Cancer Society. Often, local hospitals sponsor stop smoking programs—it's worth giving them a call, too.

There are various methods of quitting. Most people who quit do it cold turkey—stop without tapering, and tough it out through the withdrawal period, though it's tough on you, not to mention those around you.

When someone stops using nicotine, they have withdrawal symptoms. They have compulsive drug craving and drug-seeking behavior. The nicotine withdrawal, along with the habits associated with smoking—opening the new pack, removing that first cigarette, lighting it, and the feeling of relaxation it brings—make stopping much harder. That's why many people try nicotine replacement therapy or a medication like Zyban® (bupropion) or Chantix®.

Zyban® (bupropion) was used initially as Wellbutrin®, an antidepressant. When on it, many people found they lost a lot of the urge to smoke. Part of this effect might be due to the actual antidepressant action of nicotine not being needed anymore; however, other antidepressants don't seem to help that much in smoking cessation. Zyban® can be very effective. However, I tend to use nicotine replacement therapy more often, and have good results with it.

Nicotine replacement techniques that may help include patches, gum, nicotine nose spray, and most recently a nicotine inhaler.

The patch's big advantage is that it's simple. The patch releases nicotine through your skin into your blood, preventing withdrawal. Unfortunately, it doesn't give you the "hit" you've come to expect (and need).

The gum is better than the patch, in my experience. Its big advantage is that nicotine is absorbed quickly through your mucous membranes inside your mouth, so you get the same "rush" you get when smoking, only slower. When smoked, nicotine hits your brain in a few heartbeats—when chewed, it takes 30 or 40 seconds. This makes it harder for you to regulate the nicotine level precisely, so you can get too much, which causes nausea. Still, it's a useful tool, and can make a long airplane trip (or a long movie) tolerable. Using it correctly takes practice. Chew it slowly, about one chew per second, and stop chewing immediately when you get a peppery taste. Then park the gum inside your lip. The nicotine gum acts like a patch, releasing nicotine through your mucous membranes into your bloodstream.

The nicotine inhaler uses a small capsule containing pharmaceutical grade nicotine with a menthol "marker" so you can taste when it's empty. You insert the capsule into a cigarette holder-sized device and inhale, releasing the nicotine directly into your lungs. Once there, it's pumped quickly into your brain, so you get the nicotine hit just like when you smoke. And there are lots of other advantages to the inhaler.

First, unlike a cigarette, you can take a couple of puffs and drop it into your pocket. If you try this with a cigarette, you set yourself on fire—not recommended (don't make a fuel of yourself). Score: Inhaler 1, cigarette 0.

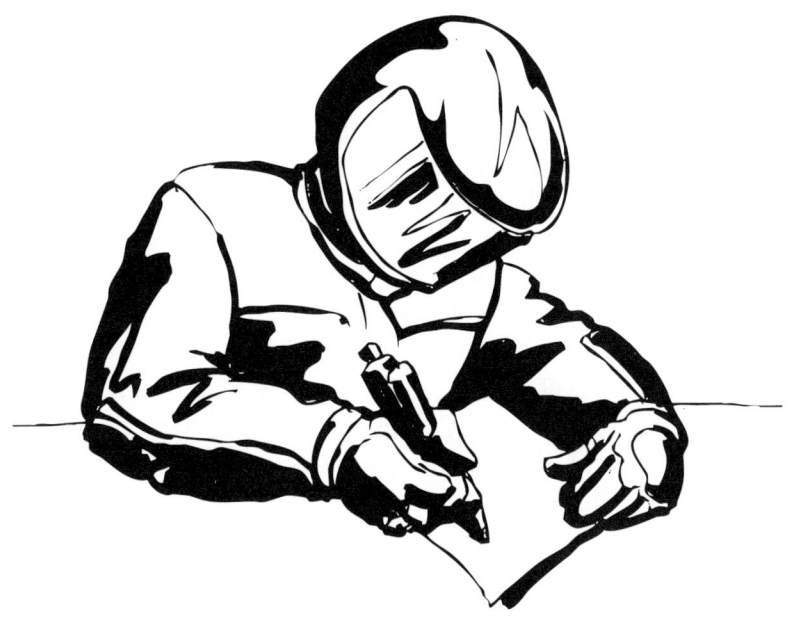

Next, you can use it anywhere. I'm typing this on a jet that undoubtedly is carrying some uncomfortable smokers. If they had a nicotine inhaler, they'd be fine. They wouldn't be wishing they could step outside onto the wing for a smoke. Score: Inhaler 2, cigarette 0.

Another advantage: There's no known health risk. Sure, you're still addicted to nicotine, but so what? Nicotine doesn't kill you, cigarette smoke kills you. Score: Inhaler 3, cigarette 0.

Okay, if you're considering stopping (again), here's a helpful technique. Don't say, "I'll never smoke again"—it doesn't usually work, probably because it's too vague a promise. It's much easier to keep a promise that you can visualize. Instead of, "I'll never smoke again," say "Before I smoke again I'll open and read this letter." Then, while you're feeling motivated, sit down and write a letter to yourself that nobody else will ever read. Be as tough on yourself as you want to be. You can even enclose a picture of your loved ones (wife, children, bike . . .) or a photo of a rotting lung.

Carrying the letter around—after you've mailed it to yourself, giving it a postmark and date—is one of the things that makes this technique so effective. Imagine you've been carrying this letter around for six months—it's probably in a Ziploc® by now—and something happens that makes you want a smoke, like the death of someone close to you, or another personal tragedy. But before you do, you have to open and read the letter. After carrying it around for six months it's more likely to affect your actions than a promise you made a half a year ago that's faded into your mental background.

The letter acts as a talisman. The longer you carry it, the stronger it gets. Imagine carrying it for five years (it's probably laminated by now). How likely is it you'll throw away five years of effort just for a smoke?

Ten years after stopping, your cancer and heart disease risk goes down to that of someone who's never smoked. Of course, if you've damaged your lungs by emphysema, they might not improve, but you won't make them any worse.

Last, here's a technique that takes a lot of guts. Print up some flyers offering to pay people $20 if they ever catch you smoking. Distribute them to friends, co-workers, and family. After that, the only way you'll be able to smoke again is to join the Federal Witness Protection Program, get plastic surgery, and relocate.

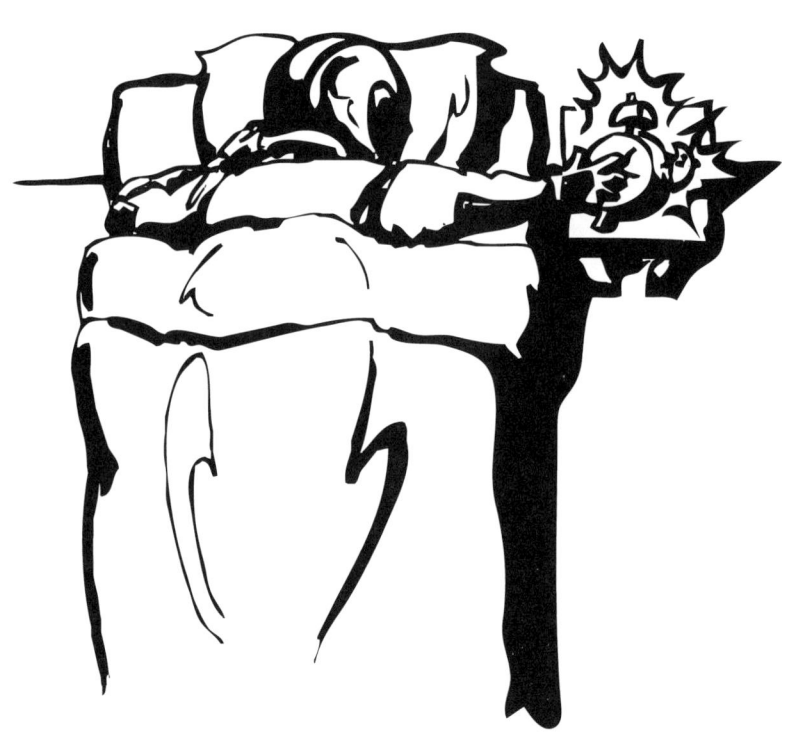

Asleep at the Handlebars

Do you wake up to an alarm clock? Then, by definition you're sleep-deprived. You're not alone—almost 50 million Americans don't get enough sleep.

The National Sleep Foundation's 2005 Sleep In America study (tinyurl.com/RLOOD) showed half of those surveyed said they get "a good night's sleep" only a few times a week or less. Of these people, 62 percent are sleepy during the day at least three times a week. And many of these millions of people are driving (or riding) while tired.

It hasn't always been this way. In 1910, people averaged nine hours a night. By 1975, it was seven and a half hours. In 2002, the typical American adult got 6.9 hours nightly. Shift workers average about five hours a night. Of course, some people need more sleep than others do. But many of us don't get enough.

This is especially dangerous for motorcyclists. After 17 to 19 hours awake, you ride as if you've had a couple of drinks, which would make you legally drunk in some areas.

The National Highway Traffic Safety Administration estimates fatigue causes more than 100,000 accidents annually, including more than 1,500 dead and over 70,000 injured. There may be more—determining whether driver fatigue contributed to a crash is difficult. Even worse is the fact that nodding off is more likely when traveling long distances on the highway at high speeds.

Fatigue can affect your health in ways besides killing, crippling, or mutilating you. Studies show a week's sleep deprivation hurts your ability to metabolize glucose, mimicking a pre-diabetic or diabetic condition. Chronic sleep deprivation contributes to obesity, high blood pressure, and diabetes. And when you're sleepy, you've got a natural tendency to eat something for quick energy, leading to weight gain.

It also causes irritability and moodiness. The NSF suggests one cause of "road rage" is chronic sleep deprivation, which also hurts job performance and personal relationships. This may lead to conflict and stress, hurting sleep. So lack of sleep leads to more lack of sleep.

Other things (besides sleep lack) can hurt your ability to sleep. GERD (gastroesophageal reflux disease) often causes heartburn at night, which can impair sleep. Common medications like pseudoephedrine (found in Sudafed® and other cold and allergy medications) often keep people awake. Of course, caffeine can easily keep people awake. Even one caffeinated beverage in the late afternoon is enough to keep me up too late.

Excessive tiredness also affects the frontal cortex of the brain, impairing memory, speech, and decision-making ability. When confronted with a need to make a sudden, critical decision when riding, lack of sleep can be fatal.

When riding, many people try using caffeine to extend their riding day. This is a bad idea. In the Iron Butt Association's Archive of Wisdom (tinyurl.com/4e6py) it's written "drugs and other stimulants do not work! If you need NoDoz® or other drugs to stay alert (the Iron Butt Association includes coffee and colas on this hot list), it's time to stop for the day and get some serious rest." Caffeine and alcohol, by the way, are two of the most common causes of sleeping problems.

Another serious problem that causes riders to be sleepy (and sometimes dead) is antihistamines. As opposed to decongestants like Sudafed®, most antihistamines (except Allegra®) cause problems while operating vehicles, even supposedly non-sedating ones like Claritin®, Clarinex®, and Zyrtec®.

Of course, when combined with poor sleep, the sedating effect of antihistamines is a lot stronger. In fact, the most common drugs found in the blood of general aviation pilots who crash are antihistamines.

Poor sleep is a leading cause of sleepiness, of course, and one of the most common causes of poor sleep is Obstructive Sleep Apnea (OSA). In OSA, the tongue, soft palate, or other oral structures obstruct the airway, interrupting sleep. People with OSA often snore, and may be heard to stop breathing on occasion. When this happens, they partially or completely wake up, preventing them from reaching the deeper (and more restful) stages of sleep. Even though you may be asleep for eight hours, if you've got OSA you don't get restorative sleep—you're still tired when the alarm rings.

When your airway gets obstructed, you get a surge of adrenaline. This results in higher blood pressure, which contributes to atherosclerosis and heart disease. Untreated, severe sleep apnea triples your risk of heart attack, increases your cholesterol level, and is associated with obesity and an increase in your visceral fat (that is, the fat inside the abdomen).

This kind of fat is a predictor of heart disease, diabetes, and hypertension. Interestingly, when people with sleep apnea get treated, they lose visceral fat; their blood pressure improves (assuming they had daytime sleepiness); and their cholesterol decreases. And so does their risk of sudden death.

In addition to daytime sleepiness, excessive snoring and choking sensations when sleeping, people with OSA tend to overuse sleeping pills. When used in the short term, sleeping pills are safe and effective. Though newer medications like Lunesta® and Ambien CR® are less likely to cause rebound (i.e., problems falling asleep after several days' use), continued use may mask the symptoms of sleep apnea, which is often easy to treat with a machine that aids nighttime breathing (CPAP or BiPAP).

CPAP (continuous positive airway pressure) and BiPAP (bilevel positive airway pressure) machines help sleep apnea by overcoming the blockage caused by the tongue, soft palate, or other mouth structures that cause OSA. Though they take some getting used to, folks who use them usually tell me that they feel much better—their daytime sleepiness, one of the major signs of OSA, is usually completely gone.

The following quiz scores daytime sleepiness. Score none = 0, slight = 1, moderate = 2, or high = 3 for the chance you'll doze off in each of these situations.

1. Sitting and reading

2. Watching TV

3. Sitting inactive in a public place, such as a theater or meeting

4. As a passenger in a car for an hour without a break

5. Lying down to rest in the afternoon when circumstances permit

6. Sitting and talking to someone

7. Sitting quietly after a lunch without alcohol

8. In a car, while stopped for a few minutes in traffic

A score of 10 or more indicates you've got sleepiness problems. A score of 18 indicates severe sleepiness, so make an appointment to see your doctor.

And don't fall asleep on the way to the office.

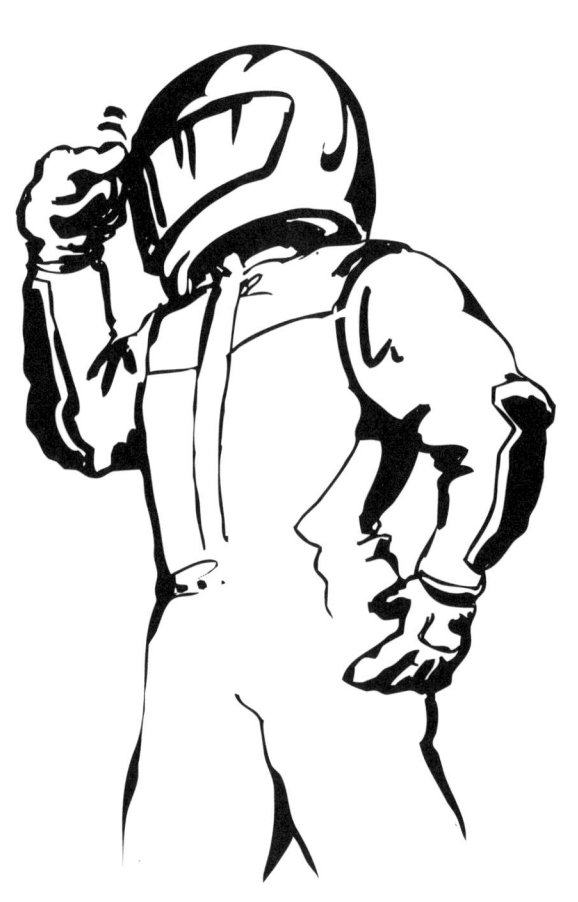

Brain Farts . . . Brrp!!

Opened the e-mail from Dave Searle, my *Motorcycle Consumer News* editor. "Doc" he said. "I guess I should have sent a reminder sooner, but we really need another column again. We ship Thursday, so we need it sooner than that."

"Uh-oh," I said to myself. "I forgot to write the column. And I don't even have a subject to write about.

"Wait a minute—I could write about memory—or memory problems."

We all have "brain farts"—we walk into a room and forget what we came there for, or we get to the hardware store without a written list and forget one of the four things we needed. Though it does happen more as we age, studies have shown that even third-graders experience memory lapses, which means that they're not just "senior moments." Aging, though, is hard on memory, even excluding things like dementia (which includes Alzheimer's disease).

Aging, though, isn't the only condition that impairs memory. Medical conditions also affect memory, including dehydration, thyroid conditions, certain medications, head injuries, mini strokes, and depression. Recently, it's been shown that being overweight can hurt memory, too.

One medical cause of "brain farts" that's often unrecognized is asthma. The brain requires oxygen to function (unlike muscles, which can work anaerobically, meaning "without oxygen").

A patient once came in complaining his memory was getting worse. As a Chief Financial Officer, he used to keep five deals in his head at once. But now, he only remembered three. He was a 30-something athlete with no health problems. I checked his peak flow (an asthma test) and it was 100 percent of normal. His blood tests and brain MRI were fine.

I asked what in his life changed when his memory started declining.

"I got a new girlfriend."

"Does she snore?" I asked. (Fatigue impairs memory.)

"No, sleep is fine."

"What did she make you quit?" I asked.

Typically, new partners will have you give up something, like beer, gambling, sloth . . .

"She put me on decaf—thought ten cups a day were excessive."

Aha. Coffee contains caffeine, which, like theophylline, helps asthma. However, we'd tested him for asthma and his peak flow was normal. I had an idea. I gave him a couple of puffs of albuterol, an inhaler that relieves asthma, and found that his peak flow increased from 100 percent of normal to 130 percent! His sub clinical asthma had never been diagnosed, but the coffee had kept his lungs open enough to improve his blood oxygen, and consequently his brain function.

One tip off that a person may have undiagnosed asthma, with the consequent memory problems, is that colds tend to go to their chest. Though this is common in smokers, healthy people rarely get chest colds unless they fly somewhere without a face mask to keep out infected mucus droplets from the guy coughing three rows back, or if they take an over the counter cold medicine like Theraflu® or Dayquil® or Contac® that dries them out too much (they're especially dangerous if folks don't drink enough extra fluids to pee clear).

Low functioning thyroid is another cause of impaired memory. Folks whose thyroid glands don't produce enough hormone tend to gain weight, get tired easily, don't tolerate cold well, are constipated, get dry hair, feel depressed, and have a slow pulse, among other things. It's easy for a doctor to screen for low thyroid with a blood test.

An overactive thyroid can cause memory problems, too. Symptoms are kind of the opposite of low thyroid—weight loss, jitteriness, heat intolerance, and a rapid pulse are often found. This is easy to test for, too, but your doctor isn't likely to test for it if she doesn't think of it.

Interestingly, your memory is not like a muscle—it doesn't necessarily improve if you use it more. In one study, a researcher divided college students into three groups and tested their memory. He then had one group do nothing, one do a lot of memorization practice, and the third learn memory techniques. Only those learning the memory techniques did better on retesting.

One of the oldest techniques to help your memory is by associating what you're trying to remember with something that's easy to recall. The association technique is credited to Simonedes, who lived in Greece about 2,000 years ago. He would associate things he was trying to remember with 25 well-known, well-remembered locations in his home.

Here's an easy way to use association to memorize ten things. First, you need to associate the numbers 1 through 10 with words that are easy to remember. These are the words I use: 1-run, 2-zoo, 3-tree, 4-door, 5-hive, 6-kicks, 7-heaven, 8-gate, 9-wine, and 10-den. For each memory word, I have a mental scene into which I place the thing I'm trying to remember. For 1-run, I visualize a racehorse running with the first object bouncing on its saddle (movement and activity in the mental scene help a lot). For 2-zoo, I visualize a pair of zoo monkeys tossing the second object back and forth. For 3-tree, I see the object on top of a Christmas tree swaying back and forth. For 4-door, I see dozens of the fourth object flying out of a spinning revolving door. Bees are stinging No. 5-hive. I see myself kicking (6-kicks) object 6. Object 7-heaven is bouncing up the golden stairs to the pearly gates. No. 8 is on a railroad gate going up and down. No. 9 has wine being poured on it, splashing everywhere. 10-den has a couple of lions in a den slashing it with their claws, roaring.

There's not much you can do to improve your baseline memory, once you've ruled out medical causes. But I find memory techniques like that listed above very useful, especially when I'm on a ride and need to remember a few things and can't pull out pencil and paper or a Palm Pilot.

Give it a try—I think you'll be astonished how well it works. And it might even cut down on brain farts!

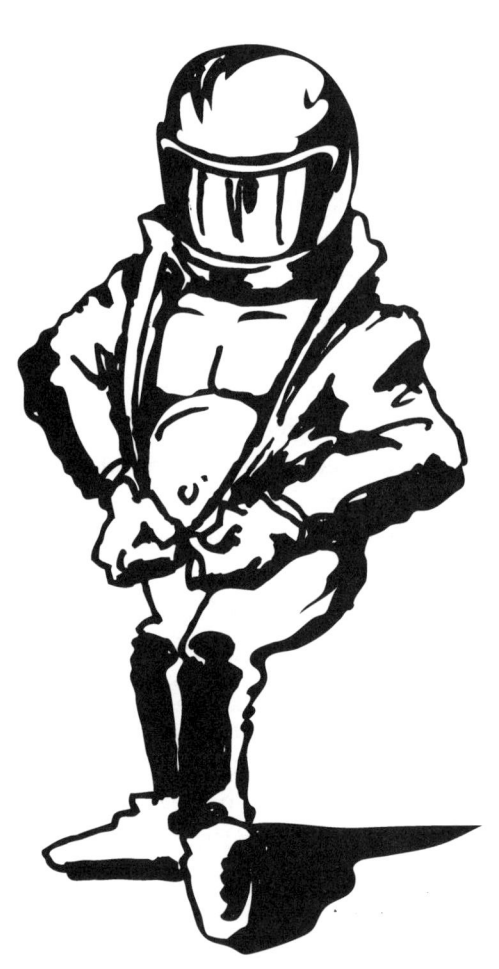

Fighting Riding Suit Shrink

My Aerostich Roadcrafter has been shrinking—and, strangely, only around my waist. My belts and the waistbands of other pants have been shrinking, too. Since replacing everything would be too expensive, I decided that losing weight would help. Unfortunately, just deciding to lose weight didn't do a thing. I realized I'd have to actually lose weight for this to work. I decided to review the medical literature, and found some startling information and interesting tricks that made it relatively easy to drop 28 pounds. Now my 'Stich fits fine. If you've noticed the same problem, the info I found might help you fit in yours, too.

Now, there are other good reasons for dieting besides fitting riding gear—better bike performance is one. Racers pay big bucks for titanium parts, carbon fiber bodywork, and the newest, most lightweight gear, because less weight equals better performance. Lowering total weight is the same as having more horsepower. I've even noticed a difference in my bike.

Bikes aside, the best reason for losing weight if you're fat is your health. Do you want to live longer? Scientists have known for a long time that experimental animals live longer when they're thin, about 30 percent below their normal weight. Here's why.

It turns out that your body handles foods differently when you're in "negative caloric balance," which happens when you burn more calories than you eat. Positive caloric balance is just the opposite—you eat more than you burn. When you're in negative balance, your body handles fat and cholesterol differently. Instead of depositing cholesterol in your coronary arteries, the fats are broken down. You can even remove cholesterol that's already in your coronaries, reducing your risk of sudden cardiac death, heart attack, and stroke. This is a big factor in extending lifespan.

It doesn't take much to change how your body handles cholesterol—it's been shown that losing a pound a year *consistently* will lower your risk of death from heart disease, stroke, or diabetes by about 75 percent. It's also been shown that men who maintain their weight at what it was when they turned 20 tend not to have the decrease in testosterone and sexual function that most men have as they age (and as they gain weight).

It's a given that overweight people who lose weight live longer than those who keep gaining. What surprised me was a recent study showing that overweight people who tried to lose weight but weren't successful lived longer than fat folks who didn't even try. It's not clear why this happens—perhaps those folks who are trying to lose weight eat healthier or exercise more, now and then. It could be that those folks who tried to lose weight achieved negative caloric balance more often than those who didn't, which helps. This directly contradicts the old saying "The road to Hell is paved with good intentions."

Folks in America are gaining weight now more than ever. You've heard about the "epidemic of obesity." It's real, and it's not funny. Obesity-related heart disease, diabetes, hypertension, and some cancers kill about 300,000 folks in the U.S. annually, and 59 million Americans are obese. So why is it so hard to lose weight? Here's my theory.

For most folks, feeling hungry is very unpleasant. That's due to several factors—both the actual, physical discomfort that's caused by being hungry, and the mental baggage that goes along with it. Many kids were punished by having food withheld. "You're going to bed without your supper, young man!" or, "No dessert for you!" This causes hunger to be associated with a lot of negative emotions, which makes it tougher to tolerate when we're adults. But I noticed something that changed those negative feelings for me.

You know when your muscles are sore after a workout? Though they hurt, it's kind of a "good" pain—you feel proud of it (at least, I do). In the same way, after about a week of dieting and feeling hungry, I found I'd lost several pounds. Great! After that, I felt a sense of accomplishment when hungry. My body was saying, "Yes, you're succeeding in accomplishing some weight loss!" Pretty soon, the feeling of hunger became self-reinforcing. After that, the weight loss got easier. And I learned some tricks from research that helped, too.

Not surprisingly, there's been lots of research on diet techniques—almost a third of the men and half of the women in the U.

S. are on a diet at any give time. A search for "diet" on Amazon. com comes up with more than 73,000 hits. So, which diet is best?

We hear a lot about the high protein and low carbohydrate Atkins Diet. Many folks have had good luck with it. Not long ago, eating a lot of complex carbohydrates (i.e., whole wheat bread vs. white bread) was popular. Some folks are on low fat diets. There's also the South Beach Diet, the Zone Diet, the Low Glycemic Index Diet, and many more.

But no matter what diet you're on, you'll only lose weight if you eat fewer calories than you use. In theory, that's simple. In practice, it's hard. (And in theory, there's no difference between theory and practice—but in practice, there is.) So what are calories? They're measures of the energy that your body can use to make your muscles move, your heart beat, your brain think, and keep your body temperature around 98.6° F.

The trick is eating fewer calories. Some diets are shown to satisfy hunger better. Eating protein tends to satisfy you for a longer time than the same number of calories from starch (carbohydrates). Bulkier food (that is, a bigger volume for the same calories) satisfies hunger better, too. A cup of raisins, for example, has about 500 calories. A cup of grapes, about 110.

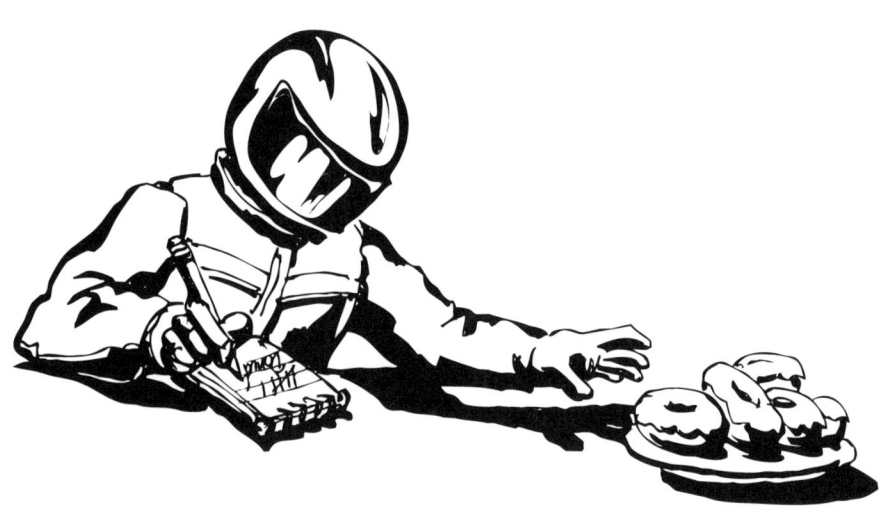

Wide Load

Trying to lose weight through exercise is difficult.

When you exercise, you get hungrier. Also, a 200-lb. person needs to walk 40 minutes daily for two weeks, at a 17 minute/mile pace (3.5+ mph), to burn a pound of fat. Though it has other health benefits, exercise alone isn't the best weight loss method.

I often recommend the Heisenberg Diet. What's that? Well, part of Heisenberg's Uncertainty Principle states, "observing a system will change that system." Now, "observing" doesn't mean "look at your food." That's the seafood diet, "I see food, I eat it"— which doesn't work. Observing your diet means getting rational about the food, and what you're doing and feeling before you eat. A personal digital assistant (PDA) or a small paper notebook (a "personal analog device," or PAD) works well. Here's why it's so effective.

Food has emotional meaning for most people. We often use it to reward, and sometimes, to punish ourselves. Consequently, eating is often an emotional, not a rational decision. Sometimes, I've arrived at work and found a box of Krispy Kremes, but only eaten half of one since I'm dieting. Not having any would make me feel emotionally neglected. Five minutes later, I'm back eating the other half. That's making an emotional decision.

Documenting what, when, where and how *before* eating demands that we be in the rational part of our minds. And we can't be both rational and emotional at the same time. Also, rational decisions are usually better than emotional ones when it comes to health. If you try writing this down:

What: one/half Krispy Kreme donut

When: 9:03 a.m.

Where: work

How (you feel): angry/sad/happy face

(i.e., bad traffic → angry)

You'll find that by having to stop and write, you'll realize, "Hey, I'm dieting. I'd rather spend my calories at lunch."

It's the stopping and documenting that helps you make better decisions. And this really works. A study comparing dieters who documented versus those who didn't found documenters lost weight over the holiday season, non-documenters gained.

Another easy way to lose weight is to stop *drinking* food. Strangely, beverages don't get counted by your brain as calories. Researchers at Tulane gave folks either jelly beans or soda every day—the same number of calories—and watched their weight. The people who got the jelly beans (solid food) didn't gain weight, since their brain counted the calories in the candy. But those who got soda, gained.

Let's say you drink a glass of OJ every morning, drink a few cans of Coke later that day, and a couple of beers after work. If you eliminated the beverages and had water (or diet soda) instead, you'd drop 20 pounds in about three months. Here's the math.

Each serving of the above beverages has somewhere around 140 calories (www.nal.usda.gov/fnic/cgibin/nut_search.pl has good calorie info on raw foods. DietFacts.com has info on brands and restaurants). Six servings times 140 is 840 calories a day that slips past your brain, unnoticed. If you do nothing else but skip those calories—no change in diet or exercise—your body will burn up fat calories at about that same rate. To lose 20 pounds of fat (at 3,500 calories per pound) divide 70,000 by 840 to get 83 days, or just under three months. It really works.

In a year, you'll be 306,600 calories down, or 88 pounds. And at that rate, a 200-pound person would disappear in a little over two and a quarter years. *Ahem.*

Seriously, eliminating beverages is a great way to lose weight. Diet soda has no calories, and tastes good, especially when made with Splenda. If you give up one soda, beer, or juice a day, you'll lose 15 pounds a year with no effort.

Soup doesn't count as a beverage because it's thicker than drinks. In fact, soup can help you lose weight, possibly because it's bulky and heavy for the number of calories it has. Yet it's mostly water. Two cups of Campbell's Condensed Tomato Soup has 160 calories. Two cups of white rice has 412 calories. If you have soup, it makes you feel full, so you eat less of the other food.

Food with fewer calories for a given volume fills you up better, too. Four ounces of mixed nuts has 680 calories; four ounces of steak, about 180; and four ounces of carrot sticks, 46. They're all roughly the same size.

One of the best ways that I found for losing weight was eating portion-controlled food. My favorites were Lean-Cuisine® frozen meals (about 220 to 300 calories), which I'd zap for dinner, and StarKist Lunch-to-Go® (210 calories) or Sycamore Farms White Chicken Salad and Crackers® (220 calories). The chicken salads were the most convenient, and pretty tasty. By eating cereal and a banana for breakfast, a chicken salad kit for lunch, a Lean Cuisine for dinner, and a handful of grapes for a snack, I could keep my daily calories at about 1200. This sounds boring, but boring helps, too.

You eat less on a boring diet. Humans are programmed to go for novelty in our diet, which is a survival trait. So, if we gorged on one food we found while hunting/gathering and found a different food later, we'd eat that, too. This increased the likelihood of surviving a long hungry spell, and helped vary the diet. Studies have shown that people eat a lot less if their food choices are limited.

Another good technique is to tell everyone your goal—i.e. 10 pounds in three months. Peer pressure helps.

Once you're at goal, weigh yourself often. Some advice says, "Weigh yourself weekly." I find daily weights help keep you honest and focused once you've lost the weight. Seeing that extra pound can provide motivation when you're tempted later.

And it's easy to resist anything except temptation.

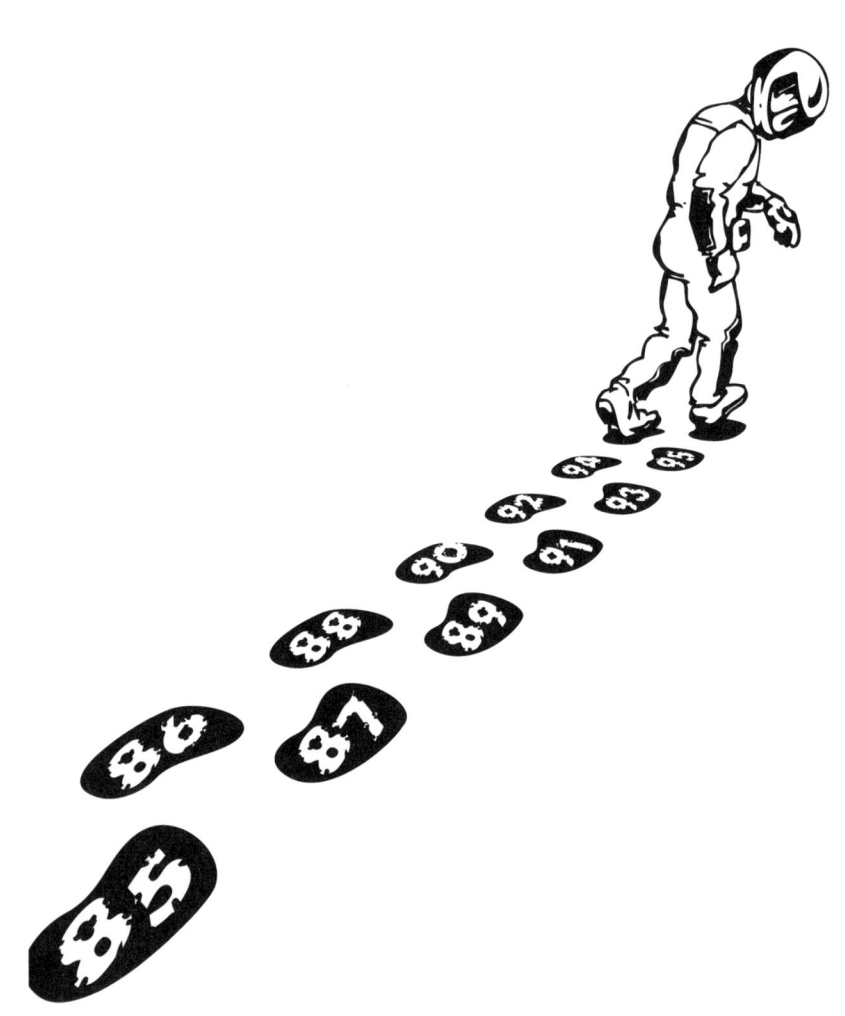

How to Keep Your Internal Combustion Engine Running

People do lots of stuff to reduce their bike's weight. My '03 Aprilia Tuono has an Akrapovic titanium slipon, saving 10 or 15 lbs. It's just as important for people to lose weight, especially if we've got more than 10 or 15 extra pounds.

Losing weight is hard (doh!). For many of us, it might be our "thrifty genes," which allow us to store calories more effectively. This helps in case of a famine, or a long, cold winter where we're stuck in our cave and can't go hunting or gathering. If we're fat, we're more likely to survive (assuming we don't get roasted by leaner and hungrier cave dwellers).

However, in these days of McDonald's and all-you-can-eat riblet dinners at Applebee's, this ability hurts more than it helps. By filling our abdomens with fat and clogging our arteries with cholesterol, the thrifty gene has turned around to bite us on our butts (and our bellies).

This load of lard we carry (think how much you've gained since you were 20—it's probably mostly fat) is linked to coronary artery disease, diabetes, prostate cancer, colon cancer, breast cancer, and hypertension. To put it in perspective, our beer belly's more dangerous than our bike.

The difficulty in losing weight has to do with how we conserve calories in "cave mode." We often don't move around as much; we consume and store as many calories as possible; and we hold onto body fat at all costs. We're like bears getting ready to hibernate. There's only one way to tell your body it's not sitting in a cave, and that's to stop sitting.

You know the feeling of energy you get after a walk (or other exercise)? That's the feeling of "mobile mode"—you're literally energized, because your body is burning fat, which has 9 calories per gram, rather than the back-up fuel, sugar, which only has 4. Unfortunately, after an hour's exertion, your body stays in mobile mode for only an hour and a half or so. But there's one way to stay in mobile mode for 15 hours a day. And mobile mode is when your body mobilizes the fat in your gut and butt so it can be burned.

If you exercise, say, five days a week for an hour a day, your body stays in mobile mode, burning more fat, for about 7½ hours—that's an hour and a half for each hour of exercise. However, after you've been exercising *every day* for about three weeks, your body realizes it's not in a cave any more. You get in mobile mode for about *15 hours a day,* or 105 hours a week. That's 15 times the fat-burning time you get when exercising five days a week. It also provides the energy you feel after exercise *all day long.*

What counts as exercise? Burning about 300 calories (for an average size person) in physical activity is enough. That's three miles of walking. Swimming, walking, running, bicycling—all work well, and the more strenuous activities allow you to burn those 300 calories faster.

You don't need to burn them all at once. I tell my patients to park a mile from work in the morning (or get off the bus or train a little early). This gives them 2 miles a day. If they also walk 10 minutes to and from lunch, that's enough to tell their body to switch to mobile mode. However, if they miss moving around for several days, their body reverts to cave mode. Also, it takes about a month, more or less, for your body to switch out of cave mode into mobile mode.

One useful device I recommend to help stay on track is a pedometer. Three miles is roughly 6,000 steps, and folks average 100 steps a minute. So if you notice your pedometer reads 3,800 after dinner, it means you're 2,200 steps (22 minutes) short. Just walk 11 minutes away from home and then walk back—you're done! And for optimum health benefit, shoot for 10,000 steps a day (about 5 miles; typically less than two hours).

Some pedometers will give you your total steps walked, total steps jogged, calories burned, fat burned, and even reset themselves every morning (keeping the previous day's total in memory, of course). Here's a good one: tinyurl.com/PD9JN.

The benefits of canceling cave mode are more than just weight loss. Cave mode has bad effects on your body due to its need for insulin. Insulin is what your body needs to open the "glucose gates" that allow glucose (sugar) to move into your muscle cells for burning. Insulin is also produced because visceral fat releases chemical signals to "turn up" the insulin levels in your body, since fat cells grow more with insulin around. When insulin levels stay high, the glucose gates into the muscles start getting used to insulin being around—and then higher levels of insulin are needed to open the glucose gates and get the blood sugar (glucose) into the muscles. This is part of *insulin resistance.* Insulin resistance is a step toward diabetes, and helps cause atherosclerosis (hardening of the arteries) in which cholesterol clogs the arteries of the heart, brain, and elsewhere. This leads to heart attacks, strokes, and aneurysms, among other things.

Unfortunately, after a number of years of insulin resistance, the pancreas can poop out. It just is not meant for constant production of more and more insulin. When your pancreas can't make enough insulin, your blood sugar rises and you then get diagnosed with diabetes. Diabetes and heart disease are closely linked. In fact, if you're diagnosed with diabetes, your heart attack risk is the same as if you've *already* had one heart attack.

Of course, having a heart attack isn't always The End. I've been there; done that; and have way too many T-shirts. I've also had more than a half dozen angioplasties to open up the arteries clogged by cholesterol. And I even use my cardiac history as justification for motorcycling. If I'm in a car, I get stuck in traffic, I can't find parking. In other words, it's bad for my blood pressure. So I just tell my wife "I ride for health reasons" (which she believes).

But now, it's time for my walk.

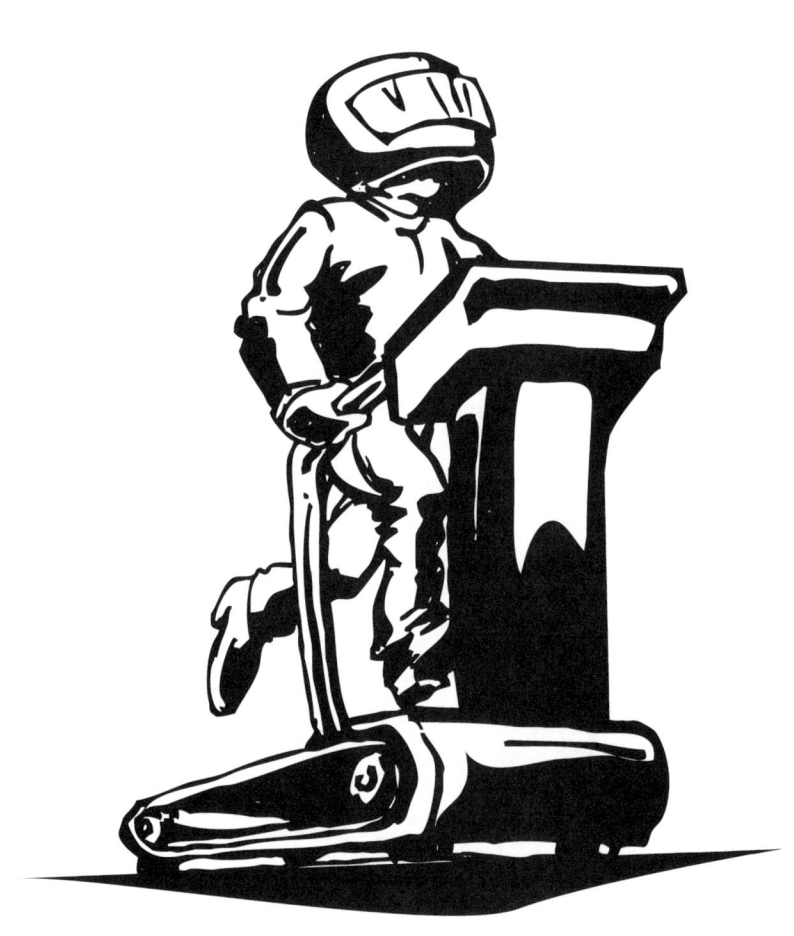

Fitness

At first, motorcycling may not seem to require much in the way of fitness, which many define as flexibility, strength, endurance, and balance. And after looking at some of the segments of the motorcycling public, I'd have to agree. But being in shape makes riding a lot safer, easier, and most importantly, more fun. The harder, longer, or more technically you ride, the more being in good physical condition helps. So, just how does being fit benefit us?

The first thing most people think of is injury prevention. Fitness definitely helps prevent fractures, from increased flexibility, greater strength, and better balance. It does this both while riding our motorcycles and in other situations. It also helps prevent sprains, strains and falls.

Additionally, better fitness gives you better endurance. When you're on a long ride, you'll get less tired if you're fit. When you're tired, you can't focus as well, or concentrate on what's coming at you down the road, or enjoy yourself after you arrive. You're more likely to just hit the sack than have fun with your friends.

Accident prevention is a big benefit of fitness—a fit rider is better able to control the bike. Tired muscles don't respond as well or as quickly.

And of course, unless you've got the skills Carol Youorski teaches (www.pinkribbonrides.com/dropped.html), being in shape means it's easier to pick up a fallen bike.

Flexibility is one of the most important benefits of fitness, but is also most ignored. That's bad, since strength without flexibility increases your injury risk.

When your muscles are flexible and stretchy, they act like shock absorbers. If, for example, you make the mistake of using your bike's centerstand on dirt and don't notice that your sidestand is still down when you rock it off the centerstand, the sudden strain on your low back as the bike falls over away from you can damage your low back. If the person doing this were very flexible, his hamstrings would have acted like shock absorbers, preventing his back injury.

Speaking of the low back: When you touch your toes (or try to) with your knees straight, you both bend your low back and you tilt your pelvis. Pelvic tilt is limited by the stretchiness of your hamstrings, the muscles on the back of your thighs. Flexible hamstrings protect your back.

The only way to increase flexibility is to stretch. Strengthening exercises, like lifting weights or using Nautilus/Cybex machines, doesn't count—in fact, strengthening muscles without stretching them makes them tighter. That's why some bodybuilders who don't stretch become "muscle-bound"—their tight muscles keep them from moving quickly and fluidly. There's a good collection of stretches here (tinyurl.com/MP3CS) and here (tinyurl.com/PKUON).

Strength is the easiest to develop. Making muscles stronger involves breaking down muscle tissue by using it; the muscle, given a day or two rest time, will rebuild itself stronger. Strength building involves resistance, either by using free weights, resistance machines (like Cybex, Nautilus, Lifefitness, Icarian, and others) or the weight of the body (as in doing pushups, sit-ups, etc.).

Building strength is usually very quick. If someone's out of shape and starts exercising, it's not unusual to see a 50 percent increase in their strength in under a month. Of course, to do this requires careful technique to avoid other injuries.

I often see folks who want to get into shape and join a gym. They skip or ignore the orientation that should be part of all new gym memberships, and end up straining or hurting something, putting a major damper on their workouts.

I recall joining the gym up at University of California, near my home in San Francisco. The trainer giving me the orientation was a very attractive Asian woman who also happened to be my wife's dance instructor. We came to the hip abduction/adduction machine, where you're seated and spread your knees or bring them together against variable resistance provided by stacks of weight.

The trainer put the peg in so I'd be lifting 40 lbs. of weight when squeezing my knees together.

"Nah," I said. "I can do a lot more than that."

I re-pegged the weight stack at 120 lbs. and brought my knees together hard.

"Ow!"

That was the first time I had a groin pull, which took about 18 months to heal. I mention this to remind others about the danger of testosterone poisoning when exercising.

The next element of fitness is endurance, or cardiovascular fitness. Typically, walking, jogging, running, swimming, or bicycling is used as aerobic exercise. You don't have to be exercising to the point of breathlessness to help your heart. If you feel like you're giving a "six out of ten" that's enough to build your cardiovascular system. One rule of thumb is that you should still be able to talk in sentences, not just gasp out a word at a time, when exercising. It's safe to do some cardiovascular work daily. You don't need a day off like you do after strength training.

Balance is another part of the fitness equation. As motorcyclists, we probably have better balance than average. And good balance is usually a sign of good fitness. One test I do in my practice is to see how long a patient can balance on one foot. Being able to do this for a minute or more is a good sign.

If you want to work on improving your balance (which includes strengthening the muscles you use for balance) a "Bosu" (bosu. com) is a great device. It's half an exercise ball mounted on a fixed, flat base. You stand on it while doing other exercises, such as biceps curls. It's possible to stand on either the ball or the base side to vary the difficulty.

Please remember your exercise routine should include balance (great for motorcyclists); strength (you need a rest day after breaking down muscle); stretching (tight muscles lead to injury—stretch before and after each workout) and cardio (basically, any activity that increases our heart rate and makes us breathe hard counts as aerobic).

Except, of course, talking with cute Asian dance instructors.

Index